CE/43.

25p

From

The Women's Press Ltd
34 Great Sutton Street, London EC1V 0DX

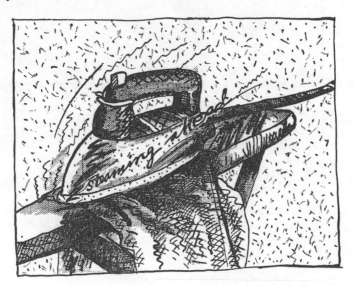

D0313091

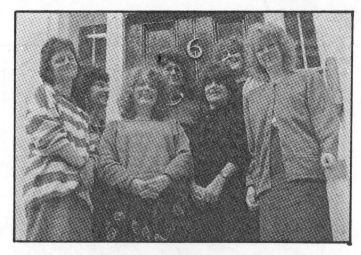

The Staff Study Group, The Women's Therapy Centre. From left to right: below – Carole Sturdy, Vivien Bar, Susie Orbach, Marie Maguire; above – Sheila Ernst, Margaret Green, Mira Dana

satisfactory meeting of the infant's needs for merger and relating. It is only when the infant has 'taken in' sufficient supplies from the mothering person (or people), when it has
received the psychic nourishment necessary to sustain psychological growth, that it can proceed towards individuating. The
taking up of a secure subjectivity occurs when the developing
baby has experienced 'good enough mothering'. Without
these conditions, attempts at separation—individuation are
based on false and defensive differentiation. Loss coming from
inadequately met needs is not a prelude to psychological differentiation but is instead a stimulus for splitting and the creating
of, in Winnicott's words, 'a False Self'[3] or in Fairbairn's words,
'the maintenance of the schizoid position.'[4].

The dynamics of the mother—daughter relationship illuminate why differentiation is such a problematic issue for
women. Very briefly, 'unseparated mothers' have scant psychological resources to draw on in terms of providing their daughters with a separate subjectivity. A mother's need for a merged
attachment with her daughter creates a particular push—pull in
the mother—daughter relationship which precludes the
daughter's having a consistent experience of being related to.
This inconsistency then means that attempts at separation are
in essence a flight from difficulties in the original merger.
Separation under such conditions is an attempt to deny, cut
off, split off and repudiate the need for mothering/nurtur-
ance, rather than the outcome of the little girl having received
sufficient supplies to take up subjectivity.

The third point that I wish to discuss, is what is meant by
nurturance within the feminist therapy relationship. It is the
responsibility of the therapist (who has, after all, set her or
himself up as available to the person in difficulty) to create the
conditions which will lead to an enabling therapeutic relationship. Individuals (most often) seek therapy because they are in
some kind of distress. They are coming for help with that distress. They seek out psychotherapy as a means to change. Psychotherapy is thus not simply an exploration of interesting
themes. It is concerned with understanding the defences and
the unconscious and conscious desires of the individual
woman; it is concerned with restructuring the psyche so that

the split-off parts can be integrated; it is concerned with dissolving the defence structure; it is concerned with restarting developmental processes that have become stuck or distorted. As Guntrip writes, 'We do not so much grow out of our childhood, as grow over the top of it'.[5] The task of therapy is to respect and respond to the adult who still has a child inside her. A child whose needs are so compelling that they prevent her from being able to use what may be there for her in an adult relationship.

Thus, for us, an imperative of the feminist therapy relationship is to provide a relationship which can contain the 'needy little girl inside'. A relationship that is prepared to receive the pain, the shame, the upset, that the client feels about her needs and her desires for nurturance. This is, however, no easy task because a therapy relationship is not about dispensing love or caring. It is precisely because the caring cannot be metabolised by the client that she is in psychic difficulties. She finds it enormously difficult to assimilate what she most wishes. She can't digest what love there may be for her. She does not trust it. She may disparage it or defend against it. She desires the contact but may be unconsciously impelled to try to undo it. The work of therapy then from our point of view has as one of its foci the therapy relationship and how it can be used as a way to take in the psychic nourishment that the client needs in order to develop. This inevitably means that the defence structure and the defences *against* intimacy become a very important part of the therapeutic dialogue. It is not that love is given, it is rather that the impediments to contact are explored. Indeed it was the strength and persistence in so many clinical examples of women's defences against closeness that led us to see this as a focus for the work. As we argue elsewhere in this collection, it is customary for therapists to see the overwhelming nature of women's desires as *the problem* that has to be addressed. Both the therapist and client may collude in a view that it is the woman's needs that are the problem. Therapeutic effort is then directed towards a restructuring of the defence mechanisms to silence those desires more effectively. In contrast to this, the intent of feminist psychoanalytical therapy is to address the woman's desires and the defences against those desires both in and outside the therapy.

SHEILA ERNST
AND MARIE MAGUIRE (editors)

Living with the Sphinx

Papers from the Women's Therapy Centre

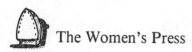 The Women's Press

First published by The Women's Press Limited 1987
A member of the Namara Group
34 Great Sutton Street, London EC1V 0DX

British Library Cataloguing in Publication Data

Living with the sphinx: papers from the
    Women's Therapy Centre.
    1. Psychotherapy   2. Women—Psychology
    I. Ernst, Sheila II. Maguire, Marie
    616.89'14 RC480.5

    ISBN 0-7043-4025-9

Typeset by Boldface Typesetters Ltd, 17a Clerkenwell Road, London EC1
Printed and bound by Hazell Watson & Viney Ltd, Aylesbury, Bucks

Contents

Acknowledgments

Early on in the history of the centre, we decided to spend a period of time together each week in which we would talk about women's psychology, drawing on our own personal experience, our work with clients and our reading of both feminist and psychoanalytic work.

This group, and its companion 'peer supervision' group, became almost an institution within the centre, around which staff members organised their working week. Some of the chapters in this book derived from work originally done in the study group, which was then developed by an individual and brought back to the group for re-discussion. Luise Eichenbaum and Susie Orbach, who left the Women's Therapy Centre in 1981, did not participate in the study groups around the book. Thus they were not able to write their chapter taking into account discussions of Vivien Bar's paper. Ultimately each chapter represents the views of the individual writer. Other members of the Women's Therapy Centre staff, and other book contributors, would not necessarily support their opinions. And there are wide differences of view on major issues even within the study group. Some members believe this to be in itself constructive, while others feel that the views expressed are too disparate and would like to return to a centre with a more unified position on clinical, theoretical and political issues.

The Joseph Rowntree Charitable Trust was particularly interested in encouraging us to spread our knowledge through teaching and writing, and funded our in-service training, including the study group. Jill Hopkins of the Trust, who liaised with us, was also personally interested, and her encouragement was especially important on the many occasions when we lost any confidence that the book would ever reach the publishers.

Jo Ryan and Julia Vellacott each made unique and valuable contributions to this book. Not only did they give excellent and extensive editorial assistance at difficult stages; they also enriched the project with their intellectual and political understanding, and their enthusiasm for what we were trying to do.

We would also like to thank The Women's Press for putting so much trust in our getting on with the job, particularly when many of us were writing for publication for the first time.

Current Staff Members of the Women's Therapy Centre:
Vivien Bar, Sally Berry, Mira Dana, Marie-Laure Davenport, Sheila Ernst, Janet Fishwick, Eva Gell, Iona Grant, Sue Krzowski, Marie Maguire, Jose Nicolson, Carole Sturdy.

Associate Members: Ellie Chaikind, Luise Eichenbaum, Esther Green, Margaret Green, Susie Orbach, Ruthie Smith, Alison Swann, Margot Waddell.

To all the women we've worked with
at the Women's Therapy Centre

The Women's Therapy Centre

The Centre is a small but complex organisation, started by Luise Eichenbaum and Susie Orbach in the basement of one of their homes. Eleven years later it is run by a staff of twelve therapists and administrators. We offer psychoanalytic therapy (what we mean by this is discussed in several of the papers) for individuals and groups, couple therapy and a varied programme of theme-centred workshops and short groups run by freelance facilitators, using a wide range of approaches, drawing on psychoanalytic theory in some cases, and using many of the humanistic therapies. (Two of the many approaches to workshops are illustrated in the papers on abortion and unlearning racism.) The Centre has an advice and information service on women's mental health issues, does specialised work on eating problems and runs an educational programme for professsionals in related fields. It has begun to see the influence of its approach both amongst professionals in other voluntary and statutory agencies and in the setting up of other therapy centres for women in Britain and in the WTC Institute New York.

Our rooms are on the top floor of the Manor Gardens Centre in North London, sharing facilities with other voluntary and statutory agencies ranging from the infant welfare clinic to Gay Teenagers. By a nice historic irony, the building was originally used as a Victorian charity run by the ladies of Hampstead for the poor women and children of Holloway, and the WTC floor was the rooming-in space for unmarried mothers and their babies. In keeping with the 1980s we are a voluntary agency, registered as a charity, and receive funding from public sources, Trusts, and fees on a sliding scale from those clients who can afford to pay.

Although far less publicly visible than the workshop and education programme, and the advice and information service, the psychoanalytic therapy and the theoretical work of the WTC are in fact the centre of its work.

1

Introduction: Living in the Question

After writing this book we realised that it dispels a myth: namely that the Women's Therapy Centre has a united 'line' on the relationship between feminism and therapy. 'What is feminist therapy?' is not a question to which we have one agreed answer, but is rather a part of a debate in progress. Some of us call ourselves feminist therapists, others think we are involved in defending what it might be, and others consider themselves to be feminists and therapists. What we have come to see is that we are in fact having to tolerate not knowing, not always having the answer to the questions raised by our therapeutic practice with women: this is both an exciting and an extremely uncomfortable and anxiety provoking experience which we try to share with the reader of this book. It is for this reason that we have called the book *Living with the Sphinx*. The content of the book reflects the discussions and debates we have had about our practice as therapists, as administrators of an organisation, and as feminists, and how we can use and develop psychoanalytic theory to illuminate this experience.

We hope that the ideas that we present will be relevant for many different women who want to understand more about women's psychology and how it affects their personal and political experience. The book offers understanding rather than recipes for changed and improved behaviour. We also hope that it will say some useful things about psychoanalysis and women but we do not attempt to give a general account of the nature of psychoanalytic theory. What we have to say may be relevant for other psychotherapists who work with women;

we also want it to be useful to the many women who work in fields closely related to therapy and who attend the weekend courses that we run at the Women's Therapy Centre; they have been important both as an audience for whom we had to prepare ourselves and as collaborators in helping us to discover how what we know as psychotherapists can be applied in other situations.

Group-life of the WTC

The production of this book reflects the recent history of the Centre, which has gone through a period of change and development that parallels those within feminism itself, and has been influenced by changes within the wider political context.

Luise Eichenbaum and Susie Orbach founded the WTC in April 1976. By the time they had both ceased to be full-time staff members five years later, the Centre was an established voluntary organisation. Their departure had a profound effect on the whole centre.

As Carole Sturdy writes in her paper:

the Centre was founded by energetic and resourceful leaders . . . who defined the organisation's aims. These aims did not have to be consciously articulated, although they sometimes were, since they were contained within the minds and convictions of the leaders . . . As in many other voluntary organisations, too, the departure of these initial informal leaders, combined with subsequent changes in the external social and economic environment, produced a need for the group to change, re-define its aims and adjust its administrative structure.

Susie Orbach and Luise Eichenbaum described their experience of using the structures at the WTC in *Inside Out . . . , Outside In*.[1]

Internally our learning has taken place in three specific ways. One has been the peer supervision group for the staff at the Women's Therapy Centre. Here we have discussed together what we were learning about women's psychology from the point of view of practice and technique. The group has shared a feminist perspective, although the routes into feminist psychotherapy were different for all of us and our group has always had some theoretical differences. The second context has been the staff study group where we have talked extensively without pressure and with great pleasure about our views on topics such as female sexuality, depression, psychological development, dreams, etc. always trying to start from our own personal and clinical experiences before moving on to reading. The third component of our learning has come from being part of the office administration – seeing what people are wanting from the Women's Therapy Centre . . . (p.8)

However generously Susie Orbach and Luise Eichenbaum acknowledged the collective learning at the WTC and recognised the existence of different theoretical positions, in their teaching with Sally Berry and later in their first joint book they articulated their own coherent view of feminist therapy. Those of us who remained at the Centre after they left, or joined the Centre later, had to work out what we thought about women's psychology and doing psychotherapy with women. Some of us already had our own different theoretical viewpoints; some were close to Susie and Luise's work but had absorbed and owned it for themselves to varying degrees; others did not really know what they thought and had not yet had to take up a firm position in public.

Faced with requests for speakers on topics like 'Women's Psychology' or 'What is Feminist Therapy?' staff members could either refuse or accept and do the necessary work. Similarly with courses, staff had to decide whether we could run them or not.

Recognising that each person had some special interest or areas of knowledge and ability, we agreed that we would each teach one session of the now established WTC weekend seminars. The commitment to doing this was based on ideas like skill-sharing and the capacity of the group to support the

4 Living with the Sphinx

individual development of its members and encompass and contain difference. In turn, some of the members of the study group felt able to commit themselves to writing papers for this book.

All of the members of the study group, during this period, contributed to the book (whether they actually wrote a chapter or not) by providing a group environment ('setting') which could contain the anxiety involved in allowing individual women to develop and differentiate (as separate individuals – see the chapter by Sheila Ernst).

Over half the WTC's existence has now been without Susie and Luise as full-time staff members; it can be difficult to recapture the anxieties felt about whether we could run the WTC on our own. Their leaving coincided both with demands from our funders for a new level of monitoring, or record-keeping, and financial accountability, and with the prolonged illness and death of one of our staff members. We also had two of our most experienced therapists on maternity leave.

At times we oscillated (as Carole Sturdy points out on p.44) 'between being a collection of differentiated adults working together co-operatively to achieve common goals, and being a collection of group members unconsciously driven to preserve their collective defences against the nameless fears aroused by the "questioning attitude"'. Carole Sturdy draws on Bion's ideas of the distinction between the former, a group working on a rational level, and the 'basic assumption' group which appears to act spontaneously and instinctively 'as one' usually behind a leader and to avoid seeking out knowledge of any kind (p.44).

When we were caught up in our anxieties we hung on defensively to what J. Chasseguet-Smirgel[2] calls the 'egalitarian ideology', needing to preserve the group illusion of unity from any attacks or disagreements. At these times we were not able to allow any theoretical differences or challenging which might threaten the coherence of the group. Chasseguet-Smirgel explains this as being a way of turning the group *itself* into an omnipotent mother; the group thus avoids the anxieties inherent in feeling like an infant in relation to an all-powerful mother.

Unlike many other egalitarian organisations which do implode, the WTC has been able to swing back into the work mode, often pulled by one or two individuals who were able to extract themselves from the group sufficiently to point out that we had to get on with the work. Perhaps the nature and commitment of ongoing psychotherapy is relevant here. The work is clearly bounded and involves being utterly reliable and regular. We have been continually pulled back to task by the need to find funding, to present our work in ways which could attract funding and to find other ways of earning money for the Centre. Similarly, in writing this book, the initial commitment to write papers based on a study programme funded by the Rowntree Trust, and later our contract from The Women's Press, has had the same effect.

Taking a group analytic model[3] which emphasises the positive and creative aspects of the group as well as its defensive, psychotic mechanisms, we can see how the realities of funding and contracts gave a context, within which the firm structures of peer supervision and study group provided a safe setting and boundaries for creative work. While at times we fell back into defensive strategies we were also able to use the group as an arena or, in Winnicott's terms, a 'playground',[4] within which each woman was able to see different hidden parts of herself mirrored, and could begin to own and use those parts. This aspect of the group has enabled us to do our work of separating; to begin to see each other as different individuals and to dare to write something down, for public consumption, which shows our individual differences as well as our shared experiences. This means that while most of the papers have been written by individuals with support and discussion from other study group members, we have had to stop clinging together in a false intimacy and feel the kind of isolation and need for a more real intimacy that Susie Orbach and Luise Eichenbaum describe in their chapter. Having different opinions and engendering conflict is something which Carole Sturdy and Marie Maguire both point to as being particularly difficult for women. For some of us this challenged our unconscious assumptions that other women, like our mothers, would not be able to cope with our strengths and might be envious (as

Marie Maguire describes in her chapter). Susie Orbach and
Luise Eichenbaum had given us a model of two women who
(while acknowledging their fears, difficulties, and struggles)
were able to say and *write* what they thought.

Each woman who wrote has had to deal with her fears both
of being envied and of her own envy. Marie Maguire suggests
that many women will have to acknowledge this part of themselves before being able to risk being more successful. As Mira
Dana and Margaret Green's papers illustrate, the questioning
of group norms may imply the risk of social isolation. They
both suggest that behind correct political lines on abortion and
racism lurks another world of irrationality which we need to
explore. In the process of preparing, reading and discussing
Margaret's paper, we have looked more closely at our own
class and ethnic origins, while in discussing Mira Dana's
chapter, we were led to reconsider the ethical issues involved
and our underlying responses to pregnancy resulting in birth
or termination.

Carole Sturdy argues for the need to reclaim the 'male'
aspects of running an organisation; in particular the need for
management. Perhaps part of differentiation for a woman
involves a reintegration of these so-called male parts. For
those of us who are therapists, dealing with the emotional
areas of life is in some ways an extension of the mothering
role, as are some (but not all) aspects of administrative work,
whereas theorising about activity for a public audience is more
commonly done by men.

Writing this book has involved us in a process which is only
now becoming conscious and available for us to articulate;
namely the process of women developing separate identities
within a group framework. Thus the writing of the book reflects
many of the issues which emerge as themes within the book.

The context of the Women's Therapy Centre

The women's movement brought 'the subjectivity of oppression, the connections between personal relations and public

political organisation, the emotional components of consciousness', into the arena of 'political thought and action'.[5] Yet among
feminists, women's mental health and therapy has only slowly
come to be seen as an important issue to be taken up on its own
terms. Feminism itself was seen as a far more effective form of
promoting personal health for women. Phyllis Chesler's
seminal book, *Women and Madness*,[6] typified some early feminist attitudes to mental health services. She showed how existing psychiatric and psychotherapy services pathologised
women, seeing them as mad and/or bad when often they were
rebelling against their own unbearable situations in the only
ways available to them. Psychotherapy, which in the US is far
more incorporated into the medical establishment, was seen as a
form of adjustment therapy, whereas women organising together politically found that personal and family changes were
often a consequence. Some of the earliest reports of women
organising illustrate this point with stories of women who had
never stood up for themselves challenging their husbands,
authority figures and the division of·labour in the home.[7] Similar accounts of the women's groups supporting the miners'
strike have been published: in a pamphlet produced by the
North Yorkshire Women Against the Strike there are several
accounts of how becoming involved in a women's group cured
women who had been suffering for years.

> I suffer from agoraphobia, and I'd been virtually house-
> bound for thirteen years before the strike started. I couldn't
> even go to the shop on my own. My husband and son are
> both miners so when the kitchen started up in the Church
> Hall at Hightown they persuaded me to volunteer. I was a bit
> nervous about the idea, but I came down and did a bit of
> washing up and got talking to the other women, and it did me
> the world of good.
>
> Since then I've hardly missed a day and I really enjoy it
> ... At first, people who didn't know me couldn't under-
> stand why. I've been to psychologists and psychiatrists and
> even spent money trying to find a cure, but this strike is the
> only thing that's done it.[8]

It seemed that Pat's emotional distress was rooted in her

social oppression and isolation, and that when she began to find a social and political way of combating this she was able to get out of her house. Professionals had not understood the nature of her 'illness' and almost by definition would not have done since they had no understanding of the nature of women's oppression and its emotional consequences. This kind of experience is consistent with the idea that the most effective way of dealing with women's psychological difficulties is through attacking the political and social causes with the dual result of both preventing future psychological distress and enabling women to 'come out' and be effective in the world.

However, it was the great upsurge of feminist activity in setting up feminist organisations and political groups which made the extent and nature of women's internal and external distress more visible. In feminist institutions such as Women's Refuges and Rape Crisis Centres some clients and workers began to think that they needed to develop ways of exploring the complexities of women's emotional experience. They began to acknowledge that this distress might have a logic and life of its own even though its roots lay in the violence and oppression women experience within society.

When the Red Therapy Group started in 1973, Sheila Ernst and Lucy Goodison recount how they 'encountered fierce criticism both from within the women's movement and from others active in left politics',[9] yet by 1980 they perceived a significant change in attitudes to therapy. (The debate however is not dead.[10])

The Women's Therapy Centre opened in 1976 and attracted many clients, both from feminists who thought the then-existing forms of psychotherapy would be ideologically unacceptable and from women who had (actually) found available psychotherapeutic or psychiatric treatment unhelpful and recognised that the WTC was saying something which they felt intuitively was important for them.

The WTC's existence and the response to it was an indication of the incompleteness of the original feminist opposition to therapy as well as the shortcomings of some of the therapy that was available for women. Psychic distress might be formed and determined by external factors, but it existed in its own right and had to be responded to in its own terms. Those of us who came to work at the WTC were implicitly taking up the question of how the unconscious might be related to the external world; and in particular what this might mean for the development of women's psychology.

The WTC has been only one part of a growing interest in women's psychology and its relationship to social and economic factors. On the one hand, there has been significant research on women and depression, relating depression in women to associated external factors.[11] On the other hand, psychological studies (starting with Jean Baker Miller and Dorothy Dinnerstein and moving on to Nancy Chodorow and Luise Eichenbaum and Susie Orbach)[12] cast light on aspects of women's socialisation which mean that women are more likely than men to express and be more receptive to the vulnerable aspects of emotional life and to be in contact both within and outside the family with the rawness of other people's psychic pain.

At the same time, within feminism there was a movement to reappraise the initial rejection of Freud and psychoanalysis. Juliet Mitchell describes this development in the introduction to *Psychoanalysis and Feminism*:

> Very recently, there has been growing interest by some feminist groups in Freud's work, but so far there is only one part of the movement that has been trying consistently for some time to turn psychoanalytic theory into political practice . . . 'Psychoanalyse et Politique' . . . Their concern is to analyse how men and women live as *men and women* within the material conditions of their existence . . . They argue that psychoanalysis gives us the concepts with which we can comprehend how ideology functions; closely connected with this it further offers an analysis of the place and meaning of sexuality and of gender difference within society.[13]

Thus starting from a dissatisfaction with any 'economist understanding of the position of women'[14] some feminists in this country have followed their French sisters to a re-examination of Freud. In 1979 *MF* was started, a journal publishing articles written from this viewpoint.

Dialogue between the Lacanian feminists and the other feminists practising as therapists has been difficult; at a series of discussions/workshops, 'Re-opening the case: feminism and psychoanalysis' in London in 1982, the gulf between the structuralist perspective and the clinical perspective seemed enormous. More recently there has been some correspondence in *Feminist Review*[15] focusing on a structuralist critique by Nicky Diamond of Susie Orbach's work on compulsive eating. Some of the problems of discussion between people who are using a quite different 'discourse' have emerged. Nicky Diamond accused Susie Orbach of being fundamentally anti-feminist because she saw her as reinforcing accepted cultural definitions and categories of women as fat and thin. Susie Orbach and other therapists at the WTC replied that they started in therapy working with the categories which women themselves used and enabled women to change their understanding and attitudes towards the concepts of fat and thin. Nicky Diamond looks at fat and thin as relational terms within a system and points out that social meaning is created by the relationships between oppositional terms within a system. Thus when fat is given the social value undesirable, thin acquires the social value desirable. Unless these values are directly challenged, using these terms is a way of reinforcing these values. As an analysis of relations within a system it is difficult to challenge this viewpoint, though equally it is hard to see where it meets with Susie Orbach's work on women's cultural use and abuse of their bodies as a way of expressing distress and protest.[16] It is not clear whether what constitutes an argument for Nicky Diamond would be a relevant point for Susie Orbach and vice versa.

At the WTC we have been struggling to develop either a common language or at least an account of what the different basic assumptions are so that we may be able to carry on the dialogue. These issues are raised in Sheila Ernst's and Vivien Bar's chapters. Continuing this dialogue seems vital, for both tendencies within feminism respond to similar questions about the nature of women's subjectivity.

So far we have been looking at strands of thought developing alongside each other within the women's movement. At the WTC we found that the recognition of our common identity as women in turn pushed us to look at the *differences* between women and how we can come to perceive ourselves as different, separate individuals. At the start the WTC emphasised the shared aspects of women's experience. The differences between women were temporarily blurred. Yet this was only a partial truth; a necessary if temporary phase. The existence of an institution like the WTC which asserts women's common identity allows women the potential to be subjects rather than objects and in turn opens up the question of how women become subjects. Yet as Eichenbaum and Orbach say, 'separate womanhood is not a category that has until this last decade received any open respect or legitimation' (p.53 below).

There is agreement about the way in which external social changes have reopened the possibility of a new conception of a woman's life in which motherhood does not have to dominate. Birth control (and more accessible abortion) have enabled us to become aware that biological sex need not determine the forms of human enterprise and pursuit, as Dinnerstein points out (see Vivien Bar, 'Change in Women'). New social possibilities take time to be fully recognised; moreover they are not necessarily accompanied by internal psychological changes. For example, Mira Dana suggests that abortion is far from being an unproblematic way in which a woman may use technology to control her own life; often it may be an expression of unconscious conflicts concerning her own experiences of being mothered and becoming a mother. The effect of such changes therefore is to make more urgent the question of the relationship between a woman's internal world of conscious and unconscious experience and her external situation.

External/internal

Several fundamental issues emerge, sometimes spelled out explicitly, at other times serving as underlying themes and points of connection between the different chapters in this book. How, the writers ask, is the internal world formed? Are our unconscious processes a reflection of external experience or are they partly formed outside a social context? Are infants born with any innate capacities or characteristics? How does the child give meaning to the differences between the sexes and how does the girl understand her own particular experience of this? In the way these issues are dealt with, there are, throughout the book, both shades of difference, and wide divergences of view.

Luise Eichenbaum and Susie Orbach's chapter on women's experience of intimacy and separation draws on a body of theory that they have developed elsewhere in more detail.[17] Their assumption is that there is the possibility of a quite fluid interchange between internal and external worlds; as one alters, so will the other. In terms of theory they see this interrelationship as very complex, although they make statements which appear to suggest a very simple, direct, an even at times one-way interaction. The mother–daughter relationship is their focus for understanding the formation of women's emotional world. 'It is an ironic and cruel phenomenon of patriarchy', they say, 'that the already oppressed shall prepare the succeeding generation for a similar fate.'

Sheila Ernst takes as one of her central themes an exploration of some of the points of juncture between internal and external during the infant girl's process of development. She looks particularly at the experience of girls in the transitional stage between fusion with the mother and autonomy, the 'twilight zone between the internal fantasy world and the external environment'. The internal world is made up of object relationships formed through a combination of external experience, and the infant's own fantasies and feelings. She suggests that it is at this transitional point, where the infant begins to test out fantasy against reality, that the mother's conscious and unconscious experience of existing social and cultural images have an effect on the girl's internal world, resulting in the inhibition of her capacity to play with fantasy and experiment with actualities. Sheila Ernst thus develops a particular aspect of Luise Eichenbaum and Susie Orbach's comprehensive account of women's psychological development, linking it with the mainstream of psychoanalytic thought through her use of Winnicott's notions of play and fantasy. Mira Dana, on the other hand, uses Eichenbaum's and Orbach's theoretical perspective to explore a very concrete transitional area between internal and external worlds: through her relationship with her body, a woman can translate unconscious process into external action, without being consciously aware of this.

Mira Dana discusses the way in which getting pregnant can be for some women an enactment of their inability to contain the unconscious longing and need aroused by the experience of intimacy within a sexual relationship. The woman may then demonstrate to herself that she is in control of these internalised infantile needs by having an abortion. This account of abortion as being for some women an unconscious attempt to assert psychological control through physical means is analogous to the way in which feminists have understood eating problems as a response to a combination of intolerable internal and external pressures. So, for instance, the woman who eats and vomits may be expressing her inability to assimilate psychically indigestible early infantile experiences, and also her conflicts about the cultural notion that in order for a woman to cope and be sexually attractive, she must hide her neediness behind a slender body.

Vivien Bar disagrees with Eichenbaum and Orbach's account of the interrelationship between internal and external experience, and compares it with two quite different accounts, those of Dinnerstein and Mitchell. Using Dorothy Dinnerstein's views, she describes a dissonance between the individual and society. Society confronts the individual as something external, outside her power to control, and part of a reality which is experienced as too painful to confront. Dinnerstein believes that both sexes maintain present gender and child-rearing relations as an external support for an internal conflict about infantile dependency needs, and that the results of this may be catastrophic for humanity. So, according to Dinnerstein's account, collusion between men and women rather than oppression of women by men is emphasised. At issue here are two different ways of seeing the relationship between internal and external realities. Dinnerstein, as described by Vivien Bar, stresses the effect of individual psychology on the outside world. Eichenbaum and Orbach, on the other hand, emphasise social forces perpetuating an unequal power relationship between men and women, which play an important part in determining psychological development. 'The relating that occurs, the feelings that are generated, the obligations rendered and sought, the fantasies and longings, are', they say, 'psychological indicators of what is possible and what is not possible within the current social order.'

The issues at the centre of this disagreement have, in fact, been a focus for discussion and controversy within psychoanalytic circles since Freud began to develop his theory.[18] In her account of Juliet Mitchell's book, *Psychoanalysis and Feminism*, Vivien Bar depicts the baby, and later the adult, as constantly engaged in a struggle to create its own world, to construct meaning from chaos. Fragments of language and image are continually worked over, influenced always by fantasy. Sexual identity is the most crucial among many ways in which subjective experience is organised.

While it is true that Freud saw the baby's psychological development as strongly influenced by the external world, classical Freudianism also puts more emphasis on biology and a concept of 'human nature' as innately aggressive than is reflected in this Lacanian re-reading of Freud's views.

The notion of what it means to be a feminist is inevitably altered once we acknowledge the strength and concrete reality of our own unconscious processes. If changes we might want to make in ourselves and the outside world cannot simply be brought about through will power and collective political struggle, then the relationship between politics and individual struggle begins to appear much more complex.

What implications do these varying theoretical viewpoints have, then, for the possibilities of changing women's psychological and social situations? Eichenbaum and Orbach emphasise that therapy alone cannot provide even a personal solution, since 'nothing short of a restructuring of social arrangements is required if the conditions that give rise to women's present psychological position are fundamentally to change'. They say that it will take several generations for this to have an effect both on women's external and internal experience.

Margaret Green recognises that the 'priority now is to change racist institutions' but that 'since oppressiveness like oppression is manifest on both the individual and the social level' she argues for a simultaneous exploration of 'early object relations'. She seems to be suggesting that when white people have done some of the emotional work of combating internalised powerlessness they will be better equipped to continue the necessary struggle in society and its institutions. She focuses on an interchange between internal and external: 'Our neuroses feed the institutions and the way oppression is institutionalised feeds our neuroses.' She also challenges the 'almost universal assumption' that there's not much one person can do, seeing this as one of the ways in which racist attitudes are culturally perpetuated.

She describes the way in which our experiences of intolerable humiliation or persecution are internalised psychologically and projected outwards as attitudes and behaviour that hurt and oppress others. As members of politically radical movements have extreme difficulty in acknowledging the bullying, domineering, persecutory aspects of themselves, they 'tend to explain the oppression in terms of external forces – economic power, tyrannical dictators, totalitarianism'.

Mira Dana also describes the interconnection between social ideology and emotional life, showing the way in which an individual woman's confusion about the psychological and ethical implications of termination of pregnancy may be exacerbated within a society where widespread killing during wartime is considered acceptable whereas abortion is seen as murder.

Some feminists are, however, increasingly preoccupied with the question of why radical political beliefs are so difficult to translate into consistent political action.

Dinnerstein stresses that not until we acknowledge and mourn the realities of loss and pain that we seem at present determined to avoid, particularly the loss of infantile fusion with the mother, will we develop emotionally and be able to act more constructively in the external world (see Vivien Bar's chapter). Margot Waddell, who has worked at the Women's Therapy Centre, is quoted as asking in *Capitalism and Infancy*[19] why, in a situation that's politically and socially and culturally changing so fast . . . the internal mechanisms remain so intact . . . Now that's where I get pretty depressed . . . For example, people's primitive reactions are not just intensifications of their stated politics; they often contradict them quite deeply, and ambivalences also make political rhetoric seem uselessly simplistic.' She goes on to say that the kind of attitudes which might be attributed to the influence of patriarchy, by some people, are, in her view, defensive against very early (and now unconscious) infantile experiences of helplessness and rage in relation to the mother. She talks about the importance of attempting to understand the relationship between these very early aspects of psychological development and wider political processes (as Carole Sturdy does in her chapter). This viewpoint does then, again, bring into question whether the unconscious really is formed within society, or whether it may actually be the other way round – that, in fact, people's psychological mechanisms, including the ways in which they defend themselves against intolerable early infantile experiences, may have contributed towards or be perpetuating social forces and political institutions.

This gives rise to an even more basic question about the extent to which the baby's development is formed in relation to her actual experience rather than as a result of psychological processes which may already be in existence at birth. Marie Maguire points out in her review of psychoanalytic views on envy, that the different accounts of its nature and origins touch on fundamental areas of controversy about the characteristics and capabilities of the human infant at birth. For instance, while Melanie Klein believes that the baby has innate instincts towards love and hate and rapidly becomes capable of distinguishing itself from other people, Winnicott sees the newborn infant as much less psychologically sophisticated, without innate instincts towards aggression or envy, and as developing very slowly, initially within the context of the relationship with its mother.

Becoming a woman

Why does it appear to be so difficult for a woman to emerge from the mother–daughter relationship with a strong sense of her own identity? The sense of having 'something missing' described by so many women is an important theme in this book, and different explanations are given for this. Luise Eichenbaum and Susie Orbach emphasise the social factors underlying the difficulties in the girl's earliest dependency relationship with the mother. The part of herself which is not fully related to in infancy becomes split off from consciousness. In order for her to experience herself as more integrated and autonomous, this 'embryonic undeveloped self' of which the woman is only partially aware, must be acknowledged and fully accepted in the present.

Sheila Ernst does not describe the woman as having this same internal split between a part of herself which has remained undeveloped, almost 'frozen' and other aspects of the personality. Instead, she looks at the way in which difficulties at the early symbiotic stage are reinforced when the girl not only has to relinquish this original sense of oneness with the mother, but, at the same time, identify with the mother's female gender. Like Luise Eichenbaum and Susie Orbach, she sees the acquisition of the capacity to mother as a crucial aspect of women's psychological development. She discusses the way in which women's ability to regress and identify in reality with her actual infant, and in fantasy with her own unconscious early childhood experiences is not, as Winnicott suggests, a state of mind that appears and then disappears, but a fundamental aspect of women's personality structures. Like Vivien Bar and Marie Maguire she describes the way in which women remain more in touch with their own and other people's unconscious psychological processes. While Sheila Ernst connects this with women's fragile sense of themselves and their tendency to 'lose themselves' in relationships with others, Marie Maguire sees this as one of the reasons why women remain more conscious of feelings like envy, helplessness and inadequacy. Vivien Bar's chapter points out that Dinnerstein connected this sensitivity to women's greater awareness of their own physical processes.

Women's tendency to be more aware of emotional vulnerability then enables men to escape into 'mastery' of the world, since the feelings they find too painful to tolerate can be projected on to women.

Marie Maguire describes the way that acute envy contributes towards women's feelings of inadequacy by preventing them from developing and acknowledging their creativity and strengths. The very envious woman fears success and competition lest competitive and envious feelings in herself or other people damage her already fragile sense of self. Like Luise Eichenbaum and Susie Orbach, Marie Maguire sees women's internalised sense of low social value as a factor that exacerbates envy within the mother–daughter relationship. She disagrees with Eichenbaum and Orbach, in thinking that boys also have a sense of 'something missing'; that infants of both sexes develop wounds to their sense of themselves as a result of experiences of rage, humiliation and helplessness in relation to a mother felt to be all-powerful. But, while boys can compensate for these wounds and for the loss of a sense of infantile fusion with the mother, in childhood and in later life, women find it more difficult to develop a sense of autonomy from the mother, and to experience themselves as valuable adults. On the one hand, power and status are associated with activities seen as male, and child-rearing, women's traditional area of creativity, is eulogised without being socially valued. On the other hand, as Sheila Ernst points out, motherhood also requires women to remain in touch with those intolerable infantile experiences of helplessness and powerlessness which through activities in the external world, and their relationships with women, men can so much more easily avoid.

Vivien Bar disagrees with Susie Orbach and Luise Eichenbaum's assumption that, from the beginning women's experience is quite different from, and much less satisfactory than boys'. For Dinnerstein, loss is the most fundamental, uncontrollable and intolerable aspect of human experience. There is no question of repairing or making up either for the loss of the sense of infantile omnipotence and fusion with the mother, nor any way of avoiding the inevitability of later losses or the reality of death itself. Before there can be any real change or development for the woman, either psychologically or socially, this loss must be accepted and mourned. For Juliet Mitchell, too, it is losses and absences and other sorts of hiatuses which are the fundamental formative experiences of mental life. Deprivation is, she says, a word used to describe the indescribable, the horror of losing 'oneself through one's own unconsciousness', so that the meaning of some part of of our experience is rendered unconscious. The other major source of feelings of inadequacy is the castration complex. This is not a sense of lack which is experienced only by women, according to Mitchell. It is, she says, not 'about women, nor men, but a danger, a horror to both – a gap that has to be filled in differently by each'.[20]

What part do fathers, or men, play in the process whereby the daughter develops a sense of herself as separate from the mother? Traditionally within psychoanalysis differentiation has been seen as being facilitated by the introduction into the dyadic mother–daughter relationship of a third term representing the outside world, usually the father. He is significant for the boy in being the person with whom he can identify while for the girl he is said to provide the love object to whom she must transfer if she is to become heterosexual. Luise Eichenbaum and Susie Orbach say that, unless the father plays a primary parenting role during the girl's earliest infancy, when her personality is being structured, he will not be able to have a really fundamental impact on her psychological development. For them, it is the quality of this earliest intimacy that is crucial, rather than anything that happens at the later stage of separation. Under current child-rearing arrangements, even if the daughter becomes erotically heterosexual, they say, she will unconsciously retain her primary emotional attachment to the mother.

Marie Maguire discusses the way in which the effects of mother–daughter envy are exacerbated if there is no external support from a father or another strongly involved adult (and in many families, even when the father is present, there is not) who can help the daughter to achieve autonomy and the mother to return to adult emotional life. She describes the way in which sex-role stereotyping limits both girls and boys, making it difficult for women to develop aspects of themselves

considered to be 'male', and the way this contributes towards
the female sense of 'something missing'. A mother's experience of herself in the external world, and her own unconscious
feelings about 'male' aspects of her personality play a vital
role in helping a girl to develop these qualities.

Vivien Bar, using Juliet Mitchell's work, discusses how each
individual will construct (consciously or unconsciously)
images of another person, that is to say a man, who must have
been involved in her conception. The idea of the Father is
always present – the child has to make sense of herself and her
identity in terms of a mother and a father. Through the discovery of sexual difference the little girl finds she lacks a penis.
This discovery is linked with very painful relinquishing of fantasies about being the centre of her mother's universe, and is
repressed and replaced by a sense of devaluation and inadequacy. Both boys and girls have to deal with the trauma of
sexual difference. But it raises particular issues for girls, since
the fantasies of devaluation and inadequacy, which are unconscious, cannot be understood in terms of social reinforcement.
Here, Mitchell is not talking about the penis as an 'anatomical
organ, but about the ideas of it that people hold and live by
within the general culture, the order of human society.'[20] In
her chapter, Sheila Ernst offers a critique of Juliet Mitchell's
views on girls' psychological development.

Different views of therapy

These varying theoretical ideas about the relationship between
internal and external, absence, and loss, raise questions about
the nature of the therapeutic relationship, the meaning of
'reality' within it and whether women's needs in therapy are
fundamentally different from those of men.

Luise Eichenbaum and Susie Orbach describe a particular
way of working, called feminist psychotherapy, designed to
address the specific needs of women. It is, they say, 'concerned
with not simply identifying the structures that psychically
make us who we are but with psychic re-structuring so that the

very parameters of femininity (and masculinity) are expanded and changed'. Marie Maguire and Sheila Ernst take up a different stance. Reflected in their chapters is a feminist way of seeing the world, but they also locate themselves much more explicitly within a framework of contemporary psychoanalytic thought. Their chapters reflect an ongoing attempt to understand the interconnections between these two different ways of construing reality. Although they relate women's position in society directly to her psychological development, and to clinical practice, they do not call this feminist psychotherapy. Vivien Bar actively dissociates herself, in her chapter, from any notions of 'feminist therapy'. She adopts a position which is *similar* to the account she gives of Mitchell on Freud. We include a discussion and expansion of some of the brief comments she makes about psychotherapy even though she herself does not give an extensive account of the interrelationship between these ideas and clinical practice, this being beyond the intended scope of her chapter.

Luise Eichenbaum and Susie Orbach criticise what they see in contemporary psychoanalytic practice as a serious overemphasis on the woman's need to separate psychologically from the mother. This they see as a repetition of the avoidance of women's needs during infancy and a collusion by the therapist with the social denial of them. They stress that the 'embryonic undeveloped self' needs to grow through a real experience of intimacy, rather than being stabilised more firmly behind defence structure as a false, conforming self.

The task of feminist therapy is, they say, 'to address the original not-getting and to provide an experience of consistent caring that can be ingested in the present. Of course this does not imply that the therapist can "make up" for the loss that the woman carries with her.' She cannot, of course, get now what she did not get then from her mother. 'However the present contact can carry the sorrow, rage, upset and confusion surrounding past unmet need while meeting the need for relating that occurs in the present.'

In her emphasis on absences, lacks and inevitable losses, Vivien Bar's views might appear to resemble those which are criticised by Luise Eichenbaum and Susie Orbach. For Vivien

Bar, the therapist's role is to bear witness, listen to the client's story and attempt to reflect back to the client what she is able to understand. It is not, however, to re-mother, or repair. There must be no collusion with the hope that the original mother can in any sense be replaced by a new and 'better' one. In the words of a contemporary psychoanalyst, the therapist is 'there to announce an absence'. The client will have to reconcile herself to the fact that the 'primary object will never be found again',[21] but will have the opportunity to grow emotionally through acknowledging and mourning this loss, and all the other absences and lacks in her early life. This focus on the therapist's role as witness does not mean that there is absolutely nothing 'real' about the therapeutic relationship, or that the therapist is cold and passive. For Freud, the psychoanalyst's 'whole being' was involved in the therapeutic process. On the other hand, although Luise Eichenbaum and Susie Orbach describe the feminist psychotherapist as making real emotional contact with the client, they, like all the other writers in this book, would agree that by definition, the relationship is not 'real' in any everyday sense. There has been much debate and controversy amongst psychoanalysts and psychotherapists about what exactly occurs or is given within the therapeutic context.[23] The issues are even more complicated for those who want to understand the social and political implications of women's experience as psychotherapists and clients. As Luise Eichenbaum and Susie Orbach point out, an emphasis on increasing women's capacity for intimacy does not necessitate an avoidance of the need to mourn past losses. In her post-abortion workshops, another form of therapy, with aims different from those of ongoing individual psychotherapy, Mira Dana gives a concrete example of the way in which both of these issues can be a central focus. While she sees getting pregnant and having an abortion as, in certain circumstances, a reflection both of women's current difficulties in tolerating closeness, and of unconscious conflicts about the early experience of having been mothered, she also stresses problems with a widespread lack of understanding of the process of mourning.

For Sheila Ernst and Marie Maguire, who, from different vantage points, emphasise women's difficulty in separating from the mother and experiencing themselves as strongly autonomous women, what the therapist in fact provides is an emotional space. Within this secure relationship the client can interact, play, project, modify and re-integrate aspects of herself into a more harmonious whole. Through this process she actually creates her own sense of internal harmony, her own 'internalised good object'. They illustrate, in different ways, the sense in which the client's perception of the 'reality' of the therapeutic relationship is inextricably bound up with fantasy.

Sheila Ernst's account implies that, since the therapist inhabits a realm between fantasy and reality, she is experienced by the client as simultaneously real and unreal. She describes a session as being like the 'transitional object' described by Winnicott (the infant's special toy or comforter), to which the client clings as she oscillates between symbiosis and autonomy, in that 'space where objects are not quite internal nor external'. This is, in fact, similar to the description given by the analyst quoted above[22] who also draws on Winnicott, saying that, like a transitional object, the analyst '*is* and *is not*. This paradoxical quality of being and not being does not take away any reality from the psychoanalytic encounter. We are, as analysts, as important to our patients as teddy bears are to children.'

Marie Maguire illustrates, with the use of theory from Klein and Winnicott, the client's difficulty in seeing the therapist as 'real' during the course of psychotherapy. She focuses on women's particular difficulties in being aware of feelings of envy, rage and destructiveness. The very envious woman cannot be close to anyone, cannot grow through intimacy, because she cannot let herself both love and hate them. Internally, she feels fragmented and divided. She can only see others, therefore, in a partial or fragmented way, as, perhaps, entirely idealised, or totally hateful. If, during the course of her therapy she can accept and piece together all her different and contradictory experiences of the therapist, as depriving and begrudging, yet also generous and caring, she will become able to see the therapist more clearly as a person in her own right, with her own actual characteristics. She will become able to experience herself in a more integrated and harmonious way, and allow herself to interact more closely with the therapist to 'use' her in this process of internal integration, once she realises that they can both survive the expression of her envy and rage.

The main differences in these accounts do, then, seem to centre around the relationship between love and hate, between intimacy and separation. There are as many questions raised as solutions offered. Does a woman need to mourn her losses, accepting that she is responsible for her life now, or does she need to be helped to develop a sense of herself before she can face up to the possibility of psychological separation? Is her major difficulty in tolerating closeness, or in accepting that rage and envy are inevitably linked with love? It is obvious that there are real theoretical disagreements and that these would lead to some differences in practice, but it is not clear whether these accounts are actually in opposition, or whether they are merely different in emphasis.

Action/reflection

These theoretical debates clearly raise important questions about clinical practice. They also have enormous implications for political action and organisation. It is impossible to campaign effectively if the underlying meanings of an issue like abortion have not been acknowledged and incorporated into our strategy. As Mira Dana points out, 'abortion is one of the meeting points of those three realities – conscious, unconscious and social'. This is not to say that we deny the importance of campaigning to maintain and improve the abortion services for women; rather it is to argue that in campaigning we cannot afford to ignore the unconscious aspects of women's lives which as psychotherapists we focus on daily. The right-wing organisations who campaign against abortion appear to have an implicit understanding of how to exploit these areas when they dwell on the difficult aspects of abortion and label doctors and nurses who perform abortions as murderers.

She suggests that some of the political slogans used in the feminist campaigns to defend abortion may actually have lost supporters by simplifying or evading women's psychic realities, and points out that shifts in social attitudes towards abortion leading to and following on from its partial legalisation have enabled women to examine more closely their conscious and unconscious beliefs and feelings about abortion.

Like Mira Dana, Margaret Green explores women's feelings about an issue which is usually discussed in terms of rights and wrongs, oughts and should nots. In doing this they both give concrete examples of the gap that exists between people's stated political beliefs and their emotional experience. Encouraged and supported by Margaret Green, the WTC, like many other organisations in recent years, has become increasingly aware of the need to look at our own racism as a part of implementing an equal opportunities policy in anything more than a nominal way.

This was not simply a moral decision; the political situation in this country has altered our consciousness and practice. Within the women's movement this need to recognise both racial and cultural differences has led to bitter and distressing struggles; yet these seem to be a part of the process of learning how to become the subject of our own stories and to develop a strong sense of our social and psychological identities. The paper on white racism is about one way of using therapy skills to work on these issues.

The approach that Margaret Green uses is based on re-evaluation co-counselling which relates individual psychological hurts to a theory of social oppression. The individual is seen as having an in-built capacity to heal herself provided she is encouraged and facilitated in this by others. This leads Margaret Green to take an optimistic view of the human being's capacity for progressive social change. While re-evaluation co-counselling encompasses the idea of unconscious material called occluded memories, the aim is to bring the hurt feelings associated with them out into the open and 'discharge' them, rather than to explore, understand and integrate the unconscious fantasy world. A weekend workshop on any topic cannot in itself resolve lifelong psychological difficulties but it can give insight into unconscious conflicts and open up the possibility and desire for individual change. Within the context of the therapeutic workshop, women may draw connections between their own individual experience and their social position; this may contribute towards a way of thinking about political action that is integrated with, or reflects, emotional life. Throughout this book the writers emphasise different factors that inhibit personal, social and political change, whether these be envy, fear of closeness, or a difficulty in facing up to the pain of losing the feeling of infantile fusion with the mother. Some writers focus on acknowledging disappointment about the lack of real radical social change, and look at why, in fact, it seems so difficult to make it happen.

Carole Sturdy shows that within organisations set up to produce psychological and political change unconscious group processes may work to maintain the status quo. She discards the very simplistic notions of personal and political change prevalent amongst feminists in the late 60s and the 70s, particularly the idea that, by altering organisational forms, changes in individual relationships would inevitably follow. In fact, as Sheila Ernst points out, it is rather that external changes create an emotional space where unconscious conflicts can more easily be looked at, understood and perhaps resolved. Carole Sturdy asks what a 'feminist' or 'radical' form of organisation would be, and looks critically at the meaning of concepts such as 'equality', 'collectivity', lack of hierarchy and consensus within an organisational setting.

As we continue at the WTC to attempt to understand the effects of the current economic and political situation of our women clients, we find ourselves faced with serious dilemmas in our role as women workers. It is necessary for us to understand these contradictions if we are to define the future of our work at the Centre. For instance, if we survive as the welfare state disintegrates, one of the reasons will be that we provide a cheap efficient service outside the NHS. Are we then, as women who accept low wages in return for control over our working environment and an opportunity to put our feminist ideals into practice, colluding in our own exploitation?

In struggling to maintain our political ideals, is it possible that we will become more 'alternative' and less in contact with the mainstream of women's experience? How can we retain some sense of control over our work while using our potential to be a solid influence on large numbers of women?

There is a tendency for those involved in the development of psychoanalytic and psychological thought to minimise the significance of the external world. This tendency to retreat into an ivory tower of emotional experience becomes even stronger as the world outside becomes increasingly regressive and difficult to influence. There is a parallel tendency for those concerned with social and political activity to underestimate the overwhelming power of our unconscious process.

As Margot Waddell says in her lecture entitled 'Living in two worlds: psychodynamic theory and social work practice',[23] 'very often we are tempted to *act* because it is too painful to think'. However, she continues, 'I'm not arguing for *in*action – simply that *non*-action may at times be the most helpful approach – not as a bystander but as someone who stands by.' She is suggesting that when action is motivated consciously or unconsciously by the desire to avoid pain, it may be 'casting the capacity for development and change, however small, into abeyance, rather than mobilising it'. If we take the space to think about our experiences, learning to tolerate any mental pain this creates, we may be able to find the most effective ways of understanding problems and bringing about change. It is particularly difficult to live with a sense of not always knowing the answers, and to retain an awareness of the importance of emotional experience as the recession becomes more severe. Solving material problems can seem the most urgent necessity.

But, in fact, as the lives of many people become increasingly filled with misery and despair, the effects of this on women become even more clearly visible. It is necessary to remember that therapy is not just the pursuit of a small elitist group. There is also a struggle about the quality of life, and therapy remains a part of that struggle.

Sheila Ernst and Marie Maguire

Notes

1. Luise Eichenbaum and Susie Orbach, *Outside In . . . Inside Out*, Penguin, Harmondsworth, 1982, p.8.
2. Janine Chasseguet-Smirgel, *The Ego Idea*, Free Association Books, London, 1985, p.82.
3. See S.H. Foulkes, *An Introduction to Group-Analytic Psychotherapy*, Maresfield Reprints, London, 1983.
4. D.W. Winnicott, *Playing and Reality*, Penguin, Harmondsworth, 1974.
5. Sheila Rowbotham, Lynne Segal and Hilary Wainwright, *Beyond the Fragments*, Merlin Press, London 1979, p.7.
6. Phyllis Chesler, *Women and Madness*, Doubleday, New York, 1973.
7. See, for example, 'Social Security and Ann Baxter' in Michelene Wandor (ed.), *The Body Politic*, Stage One, London, 1972.
8. Pat Castleford in *Women Against the Strike*, North Yorkshire Women Against the Strike Group, 1984-5, p.61.
9. Sheila Ernst and Lucy Goodison, *In Our Own Hands*, The Women's Press, London, 1981, p.6.
10. See *Trouble and Strife*, nos 3 and 4, 1984.
11. M.M. Weissman and E.S. Pankel, *The Depressed Woman: a study of social relationships*, University of Chicago Press, Chicago, 1974; and their more recent work published in 1980 and 1984.
12. Jean Baker Miller, *Towards a New Psychology of Women*, Penguin, Harmondsworth, 1978; Dorothy Dinnerstein, *The Rocking of the Cradle*, Souvenir Press, London, 1978; Nancy Chodorow, *The Reproduction of Mothering; psychoanalysis and the sociology of gender*, University of California Press, Berkeley, Cal., 1978; Luise Eichenbaum and Susie Orbach, *Understanding Women* (an expanded version of their earlier publication, *Outside In . . . Inside Out*), Penguin, Harmondsworth, 1985.
13. Juliet Mitchell, *Psychoanalysis and Feminism*, Penguin, Harmondsworth, 1975, p.xxii.
14. Juliet Mitchell, *Women: the longest revolution*, Virago, London, 1984, p.18.
15. N. Diamond, 'Thin is the feminist issue', *Feminist Review* 19: Spring '85. pp.23-6. Letters from Susie Orbach and the

'Eating Problems' Supervision Group at the WTC in *Feminist Review*, 21: Winter '85, p.56. Thanks to Susie Orbach for access to unpublished correspondence in this debate.

16. See Susie Orbach's most recent work, *Hunger Strike*, Faber and Faber, London, 1986.

17. Eichenbaum and Orbach, *Understanding Women*.

18. For a fuller discussion of these issues in recent publications, see Janine Chasseguet-Smirgel and Bela Grunberger, *Freud or Reich*, Free Association Books, London, 1986; a critique of this book by J. Kovel, 'Why Freud or Reich?' in *Free Associations*, no. 4, 1986; B. Richards (ed.), *Capitalism and Infancy*, Free Association Books, London, 1984; and R. Banton, P. Clifford, S. Frost, J. Lousada and J. Rosenthall, *The Politics of Mental Health*, Macmillan, London, 1985.

19. C. Lasch and discussants, 'Family and authority' in B. Richards (ed.), *Capitalism and Infancy*, pp.30-31.

20. Juliet Mitchell, *Psychoanalysis and Feminism*, p.xvi.

21. G. Kohon (ed.), Introduction, *The British School of Psychoanalysis: the independent tradition,* Free Association Books, London, 1986, p.517.

22. See the section entitled 'Counter transference: an independent view', and other essays in Kohon (ed.), *The British School of Psychoanalysis*.

23. M. Waddell, 'Living in two worlds; psychodynamic theory and social work practice', unpublished Pam Smith Memorial Lecture 1985.

2
Questioning the Sphinx: an experience of working in a women's organisation

> I know of no experience that demonstrates more clearly than the group experience the dread with which a questioning attitude is regarded.[1]

In this article I want to look at my own 'group experience', that of working in a 'radical' women's organisation: radical not only in regard to the nature and goals of its work, but also in the way it carries out that work, its internal organisation and structure. In this article I question what is meant by a 'radical' or 'feminist' form of organisation, and suggest that the work of Bion on groups, as well as the work of other theorists such as Isabel Menzies, Elliot Jaques, and Otto Kernberg,[2] can be helpful in understanding the group processes that occur, particularly in work groups of a radical nature.

Bion, in the work from which the above quotation is taken, is writing about a psychotherapy group, a small group with no formal structure, apart from a regular time and place of meeting, and no explicitly defined task. Anyone who has had experience of such a group will know the feeling of 'dread' which he is talking about. For those who have not had direct experience of such a group, the idea of 'group therapy' has now almost as much of a place in popular mythology as the cartoon and movie version of the impassive psychoanalyst and his couch, an idea much influenced by Hollywood's picture of the encounter group, Marin County Style, whose members either scream sexual taunts and hatred at each other, or else cling to each other and cry. It is, simultaneously, both a place of longed-for community and comfort, and of dreadful danger, where we feel we may be torn apart. It is, in fantasy, a place where anything might happen. The group comes to represent, in Bion's words, 'the Sphinx, the enigmatic brooding and questioning Sphinx, from whom disaster emanates'. The group, sitting in a circle, becomes a concrete symbol of 'zero', the possibility of disintegration, that absence of an answer, which we fear and do our best to avoid.

The Women's Therapy Centre is a continually changing and, up to now, expanding organisation. It now employs two full-time administrative workers, a full-time information worker and ten part-time psychotherapists, one of whom also co-ordinates the Centre's work on eating problems. During the three years that I have worked at the Centre as an administrative worker, the group has been engaged, more or less explicitly, in a process of defining, sometimes re-defining, its overall aims and objectives as an organisation. Sometimes this process has felt a great deal like questioning an inscrutable Sphinx, trying to decipher her riddles, and at the same time learning to tolerate the anxiety, or dread, which such a state of uncertainty generates. Like many other voluntary organisations, the Centre was founded by energetic and resourceful leaders, a 'creative couple' who defined the organisation's aims. These aims did not have to be consciously articulated, although they sometimes were, since they were contained within the minds and convictions of the leaders. Any doubts could, in the last analysis, be referred to them for guidance or resolution. As in many other voluntary organisations, too, the departure of these initial informal leaders, combined with subsequent changes in the external social and economic environment, produced a need for the group to change, re-define its aims and adjust its administrative structure. The Women's Therapy Centre has attempted to do this by consensus, with no formally acknowledged leadership, an enormously difficult task.

The Centre's overall aims, their context and history, have been described in the Introduction to this book. In this chapter I want to examine, from my own experience as an administrator, that aspect of the Centre's aims that is particularly concerned with organisation and structure. One of the aims of the Centre, since I have been there, whether expressed or not, has been that its internal structure and culture should reflect or embody the group's feminist values. In other words, that we were to express our feminist perspective not only in what we did as a group, but also in how we did it. This aim, of course, begs a great many questions. Is there any consensus, to begin with, either within or outside the Women's Therapy Centre, about what 'feminist values' are? How are they to be developed and by whom? Can they be applied to organisational forms? Are they necessarily congruent, or can they be contradictory? Just these few questions are enough to indicate some of the difficulties.

The Centre's structure, since I joined it, has been a collective one. Although no formal decision was ever taken at any point in the group's history to 'go collective', it nevertheless now operates as though it were one, for all practical purposes. All policy decisions are made at monthly staff meetings by the whole staff group and as far as possible by consensus. Only in exceptional cases are decisions reached through a vote (for example, when a quick decision needs to be made on a relatively minor issue). Otherwise, if there is disagreement on a more important issue, the decision is deferred so that the conflict of opinion can be discussed further until some form of compromise can be reached. Although responsibility for planning different areas of work, for example workshops or courses, can be delegated to specific sub-groups, the final decision on whether, or how, these plans are put into practice, rests with the staff group as a whole. As well as working collectively, the Centre aims also to be self-managing. Although required, as a charity, to have trustees not employed by the Centre, these trustees do not act strictly as a management committee. Their role is more that of consultants, offering advice or support to the group when called upon. Workers at the Centre, both therapists and administrators, have effective control, collectively, over their work and working conditions although trustees of course have a legal right of veto.

Another aspect of the Centre's structure is that it aims to be non-hierarchical. Although it is recognised that workers at the Centre have different levels of experience and expertise, which gives them more or less *personal* authority in relation to different tasks, there is no formal power or authority attached to any *role*. For example, the Centre does not have a manager. Similarly, it does not employ anyone purely as a secretary or filing clerk, although these tasks generally fall to the administrative workers as one aspect of their work. This non-hierarchical organisation is underpinned by its policy of paying all workers, whether administrators or psychotherapists, full-time or part-time, employees or sessional workers, the same hourly rate. Although neither policy has rarely, if ever, been questioned while I have been a member of the group, it is not clear whether that is because their feminist nature is so much taken for granted that to do so threatens the basic identity of the group, or whether it is because they are a mechanism for avoiding feelings of envy and competition which might otherwise arise.

As an abstract ideal, collective self-management of an enterprise seems so self-evidently desirable to those of us who grew up steeped in the libertarian culture of the 1960s and 1970s that it is hard to criticise or assess objectively. It has its roots in the ideals of democracy itself and, more recently, in those of socialism, anarchism, syndicalism and of course the co-operative movement. But for the generation of those women who make up the majority of workers at the Centre, the ideal really entered our political consciousness via the 'second wave' of feminism of the late 1960s. As Sheila Rowbotham has put it, this was a time when 'it was assumed that your politics were communicated not only through what you said, but in what you did and how you did it'.[3] The utopian future that I, amongst others, envisaged at that time was one in which the division between mental and manual labour would have been eradicated, and where all members of society would be actively involved in its planning and decision-making, whether through local soviets, neighbourhood committees, workers' co-ops, or whatever. However, those of us involved in feminist and libertarian politics were motivated not simply by a desire to build a particular kind of future, but also by a need to transform the present. We attempted to build the kinds of political organisations, even have the kinds of personal relationships, which would prefigure the society we desired in the future. The

structure of the women's liberation movement itself, as a loose
federation of autonomous, self-governing groups, with no central committee, 'leaders' or united policy, is a prime example of
this prefigurative politics, in which 'ends' and 'means' are not
seen as separate, nor the distinction seen as useful. However, I
do not want to explore here the implications of such a structure for a political movement, interesting though that is. This
has been done elsewhere, especially in *Beyond the Fragments*
(see note 3, p.48). What I want to consider is what happens
when a feminist group takes that structure from the political
context in which it was developed, and transplants it into a
very different kind of context, say that of a voluntary organisation providing a service to the community. Such a structure
acquires a completely different meaning in the process of trans-
plantation. For example, 'collective self-management' has
very different implications in the different contexts of, say, a
local women's consciousness-raising group, and a children's
day nursery. The aim of the former is to meet its own needs
without any investment from outside, whereas the latter's aim
is to meet other people's needs with other people's money. Put
simply, different tasks require different organisational forms.
Not to recognise this would be to make a fetish of a particular
kind of structure, such as the collective, as though it had an
abstract ideological purity whose magical properties could
guarantee success. A recent book, *What a Way to Run a Railroad*, describes the thinking behind the assumption that there
is a 'correct' form of internal politics and the wholesale rejection of 'bad' bureaucratic forms:

> Since libertarians wish to model themselves neither on capi-
> talism nor the so-called socialist states, the industrial form
> of organisation with which they are associated [bureaucracy]
> is rejected for all situations. In reaction, fully democratic,
> informal, non-hierarchical organization becomes the model
> for *all* cases and contexts. Thus we have the replacement of
> one rigid decontextualized dogma of organization by a dif-
> ferent one, with a different *content*, but an equally rigid and
> decontextualized form . . . The assumption is that as long as
> we fight in the right *way* we are bound to win. From here it is

only a short step to thinking that it doesn't matter if we win, as long as we've played the game in the right spirit.[4]

For the paid employees of radical organisations it matters very much if they 'win' in achieving at least their first objective of surviving as viable organisations. Which is not to advocate a position of complete and cynical pragmatism, but simply to point out that pragmatic considerations also have a part to play when people's livelihoods are at stake.

Not only is it impossible to prescribe one 'correct' structure for all organisations, it is also impossible to prescribe one 'correct' structure for all the different activities *within* one organisation. Charles Handy, in *Understanding Organizations*, proposes that within organisations activities can be divided roughly into four sets: *steady state*, or routine jobs, like the accounting system, secretarial system and record-keeping; *innovation*, which is developmental and directed to changing what the organisation does or the way it does it; *breakdown/crises*, the part of the organisation that deals with crises originating both within and outside the organisation; and *policy*, which sets priorities, establishes standards, allocates resources and decides on action. Each of these sets of activities has its own different and appropriate culture, structure, forms of power and influence. 'Organizations that are *differentiated* in their cultures', says Handy, 'and who control that differentiation by *integration* are likely to be more successful'.[5] In other words, there are no simple, reductive solutions to the problem of structure, there is no blanket answer. What is important is that the culture and structure of each set of activities should be appropriate to its task. Which means defining the different kinds of tasks co-existing within an organisation, and not allowing the culture appropriate to one sort of activity to swamp all the others. Handy's illustration of a preferred culture crowding out another more appropriate one, will be familiar to many workers in small, radical organisations:

A lot of individuals enjoy the management of breakdown. Power-oriented, but in no position to direct policy, they get a real sense of achievment from dealing with crises. In many organizations, particularly small ones, activities which should be programmed, routinized, systematized, are in fact dealt with on an *ad hoc* crisis basis because that is the individual's preferred culture . . . It is pleasant to be busy. A deteriorating steady state produces lots of business.

(p.200)

To complicate the picture further, the balance of activities and cultures within an organisation will also shift over time, changing its emphasis. In a recent article on voluntary organisations, or 'Volorgs' as he calls them, Handy identifies three main types and argues that many of their problems arise from confusions, in which methods appropriate to one type are extended – often unconsciously – into another.[6] The three varieties that he identifies are the *Mutual Aid* Volorg, started by a group of people coming together to support each other in a common problem; the *Service* Volorg, where the emphasis is on providing help to those in need; and the *Campaigning* Volorg, where a cause, rather than a problem unites people in attempting to raise consciousness, change laws or influence policies. The three types have different cultures and require different structures; the Campaigning Volorg is *led*, the Service Volorg is *managed*, while the Mutual Aid Volorg is *served* (by a secretary of the group). The problem is, however, that most Volorgs change from one type to another, and many are a mixture of the three varieties. What Handy is again arguing for here is a more analytic, diagnostic approach to organisation, and a readiness to acknowledge differentiation, both internally and over time.

Handy's analytic approach can be very useful in understanding some of the difficulties experienced at the Women's Therapy Centre, and I suspect in many other radical organisations. The balance of activities at the Centre has changed considerably since it began, whereas the consciousness of these changes has lagged behind them somewhat so that appropriate structures have been slow to develop. For example, the Centre has always been a mixture of a Mutual Aid, Service and Campaigning organisation, but the relative importance attached to each of these activities has changed. When it began, the campaigning aspect of its work was considered by the founders of major importance, with mutual aid next, in terms of study and peer supervision, and then, last, the provision of a service of psychotherapy. The provision of psychotherapy has, of course, always been considered important, but it was not, at the beginning, seen as the primary aim of the organisation. Appropriately enough for a mainly campaigning organisation, in Handy's terms, the Centre was led in its early days by its two founders whose 'rhetoric, argument and charisma' (Handy) carried the day. When the two founders left, the need for mutual aid amongst those who remained, in coping with their new responsibilities, was uppermost for a time, to be succeeded by what is now the main work of the Centre: the provision of a certain kind of psychotherapy service, with other activities secondary to that. While this greater emphasis on service provision produces a correspondingly greater need for effective management, this need not be at the expense of the other activities of the Centre. However, in any organisational change there is always an anxiety that a new culture will swamp all the others and take over. In the Women's Therapy Centre this fear is sometimes expressed about 'admin': that if the office workers had their way, theirs would be the major work of the Centre, with psychotherapy very much in second place.

The vagueness with which the term 'admin' is defined at the Centre, and perhaps in other similar organisations, can increase the threat it is felt to pose. It can feel like an amorphous mass of activity which would spread like a cancer if allowed to go unchecked. Yet an antidote to this fear, which is to define the various functions of 'admin' more precisely, is avoided, presumably because it would lead to a recognition of difference which we find equally hard to acknowledge (for reasons given below). The term 'admin' is in fact used to cover a range of activities, from providing secretarial support, to giving advice and information over the phone, to what is usually called 'management' in other organisations, that is, clarifying organisational goals and working out strategies for reaching them. What function does this vagueness about the nature of 'admin' serve? First, it allows a radical organisation, such as ours, to believe that it does not require management as such. This belief is reinforced if the group calls itself 'self-managing', which can denote that the group does not recognise management as a necessary skill at all, but as something that anyone can do as a sort of sideline to their real work. It may vaguely be conceived of as 'running the Centre', and in practice consist of responding to emergencies as they arise, and generally 'muddling through'. The reluctance to admit the need for management is, I suspect, widespread in radical organisations, and is one cause of the suspicion with which 'admin' is regarded. As Landry *et al*. put it:

> Management is conceived variously as what the enemy does: as a set of techniques which are used to stabilize hierarchical regimes; as a form of rationalization; or as intelligence which should belong with the labour process but which, in its managerial form, is wielded from above as a controlling set of constraints on the debased and 'de-skilled' activities of modern work. Management is identified with autocratic authority and then dismissed out of hand.[7]

Secondly, vagueness about the nature of 'admin' allows the 'admin' workers themselves to avoid recognising the fact that their work may require different systems and a different culture from that prevailing in the organisation as a whole. This may be especially true in a women's group, where differences are harder to acknowledge. For example, the prevailing work culture at the WTC is closest to what Handy describes as a 'Person culture':

> In this culture the individual is the central point. If there is a structure or an organization it exists only to serve and assist the individuals within it. If a group of individuals decide that it is in their own interests to band together in order the better to follow their bents, to do their own thing, and that an office, a space, some equipment or even clerical and secretarial assistance would help, then the resulting organiz-ation would have a person culture . . . The kibbutz, the commune, the co-operative, are all striving after the person culture in organizational form . . . Individuals with this orientation are not easy to manage.[8]

The necessity for other kinds of cultures, such as Handy's

'steady state' culture for routine tasks, governed by rules and procedures, is resented in an organisaton like the WTC, and tacitly ignored, because everyone really wants to be working together in the same kind of culture, with no differentiation. This may not be consciously expressed. Instead, what often happens is that these more routine, unglamorous tasks (such as keeping client records and statistics) get neglected or, when a backlog accumulates, farmed out to a freelance worker outside the collective (often for a lower rate of pay). A third advantage of a vague term such as 'admin', particularly within a women's organisation, is that it is gender-neutral, unlike 'managerial' with its 'masculine' connotations, and 'secretarial' with its more 'feminine' ones. Renaming can allow us to overlook the necessity of both types of function, particularly the more 'masculine' one in a feminist organisation set up in opposition to the 'male' way of doing things. Anyone taking on a management role, part of which consists in exerting controls, can come to be seen as the 'enemy within', whose feminism thereby becomes suspect.

There are real problems involved in using the adjective 'feminist' to describe anything other than women, or female active subjects. It is hard to see what meaning the term 'feminist' can have when used to describe an organisational structure, other than that it means that it is the sort of organisational structure which particular feminists preferred to adopt, for particular reasons at a particular point in their history. Used in any other way, it is in danger of degenerating into an implicit value judgment, closing off all discussion. There is nothing inherently 'feminist' about any one organisational structure. Used in this way, the term 'feminist' is like a flag stuck into a cluster of words or concepts to warn the unwary not to question them too deeply. The term 'feminist' can suffer the same fate of being decontextualised as the term 'collective' and 'bureaucracy'. It can become a sort of dogma, unconsciously assumed to mean the same thing in very different situations. For example, the goal of collective self-management may be a 'feminist' one in the context of a conscious-raising group, or a self-help group since it is the structure that can most effectively express the (feminist) aspirations of the women concerned. It is not, however, necessarily 'feminist' when adopted by a voluntary organisation set up to meet women's needs, since it offers no means for those women concerned as users to express their demands (through a management committee, for example).

The issue of accountability is a difficult one for all feminist professionals, and particularly for feminist psychotherapists, because of the nature of their work and their relationship with clients. Even the use of the term 'client' by the WTC, instead of the term 'patient', more conventional in psychotherapy, is an acknowledgment of this difficulty. Presumably a 'client' is more of a consumer, defining her own needs and employing a professional to meet them, than a 'patient' whose needs are defined for her by the professional in whose care she places herself. This act of renaming, though it may once have been motivated by the Centre's desire to disclaim the sort of power inherent in the doctor–patient relationship, does not necessarily do so (even if that were desirable). It certainly does not guarantee that the Centre as an institution will be more responsive to the needs and priorities of the women in the community whom it serves, although that, presumably, is what a service set up by feminists aims to do.

The problem, though, with psychotherapy is that the demand for it is now great, growing, and potentially infinite. This growth in demand in recent years has led to a corresponding increase in supply, in the private sector. In other words, in this sector, the market is playing its usual role of regulating supply and ensuring that consumer demand is met. In the public sector, of course, things are different. Although the demand for therapy, in this sector, from women who cannot afford private fees, has also grown, supply has remained relatively static. The WTC, therefore, like other similar agencies, is continually faced with the problem of how to ration out its woefully inadequate resources. And the rationing of resources in the public sector involves, of course, political choices. Some of the difficult choices potentially facing the WTC are, for example, about whether the emphasis should be upon providing unlimited psychotherapy to a relatively small number of women, or on offering more limited contracts, say for two years, to greater numbers. What proportions of different services should be offered? Should there be more groups or more individual therapy? Or equal amounts of both? What account should be taken of the therapists' own preferences for different ways of working? All these questions are not simply professional, but political questions for an organisation which describes itself as 'feminist'. They cannot be ducked by arguing that there should be increased resources. Of course we must argue for more resources, but however great these are, they will always be finite and never enough for social needs. In other words, however great our resources, there will always be the need to decide priorities. The political question then is: '*Who* decides the priorities?' or, at the very least, 'Who should be consulted when deciding priorities?' It is the answers that an institution gives to these questions, as well as the content of its work, which determine its political complexion, rather than the political orientation of individual staff members.

The concept of 'accountability' can itself be decontextualised or used simplistically. Like the notions of the 'collective', 'non-hierarchical organisation', and even 'feminist', it needs to be looked at analytically, and in relation to the task undertaken. The form of accountability appropriate to a local authority, for example, will be different from that appropriate to a professional service. Obviously, psychotherapists cannot be elected by popular vote and risk the sanction of losing their seat if they fail to keep their manifesto promises. 'Accountability' does not imply that professionals do not have particular skills and that everything can be run by popular democratic vote and public meetings. Professionals offering a particular service are likely to be, in fact, more skilled and/or objective in their area than users. They are, therefore, likely to be vulnerable to the envy of their clients. Psychotherapy professionals are, perhaps, particularly vulnerable in this way, not only in relation to users, but also to others in the 'caring' professions, who may be needy themselves and who, because they feel themselves to be working under considerable pressure and stress, are envious of the working conditions they see therapists as enjoying, the time and thought they can give to their clients. The practice of psychotherapy itself is also constantly under attack from a wider public who question its value and use. In addition, feminist psychotherapists in particular face political criticism from some sections of the Left and from those feminists who are anti-professional. In the circumstances, there are good reasons for an organisation like the WTC to feel the need to protect itself from outside 'interference'. However, despite all these difficulties, the stubborn fact remains that the WTC, identifying itself as an organisation of feminists, has to confront the issue of accountability in some way with the 'questioning attitude' referred to at the beginning of this article. The difficulties simply form the context within which that questioning must take place.

The issue of the accountability of professionals raises questions about the exact position occupied by non-professionals working within an organisation which describes itself as a collective. At the WTC it is assumed that all policy decisions are made by the collective as a whole. 'Policy', however, is another very broad term whose meaning alters according to the context. It spans questions which are both obviously 'political', such as whether the Centre should send a speaker to a women's group in South Africa, and those which are amenable to both a political and professional interpretation, such as whether, for example, more limited-term psychotherapy contracts are needed at the Centre. In the first type of decision, distinctions between professionals and non-professionals are irrelevant: all members of the group can participate equally as individuals and as workers. The second type, however, is both a political question about the allocation of limited resources in response to overall need, and a professional question about what is the 'best' form of treatment for individual clients. In the example given of a discussion about the type of therapy contracts to be offered by the Centre, it is unclear to me, as an administrative worker, where I should locate myself. As an administrative worker I am likely to have more contact with, and awareness of, the daily outside demand on the Centre from individual women and from other agencies, than psychotherapists have. I am often in the role of gatekeeper at the Centre, saying 'No' to most of the demands made upon us, which can be felt as overwhelming at times. In the past it has often been the administrative workers, therefore, who have argued for increasing the accessibility of the Centre, or for rationing resources, through for example offering a drop-in facility or more medium-term contracts. Unless, however, these proposals can be shown to express the demands of users, and the Centre has given a prior commitment to take these demands into account, the proposals of the administrative workers can easily be overruled as personal opinions. My views, in this case, do not have any particular legitimacy since they are not necessarily representative of anyone but myself. This becomes glaringly obvious in any discussion on the needs of black women in the community, since none of the workers at the Centre is black, an example of the way in which equal opportunities issues, while of absolute importance in themselves, can also serve as a sort of litmus test for other aspects of an organisation's practice. Internal democracy and collective-working practices, within a voluntary organisation, cannot be a substitute for external consultation and accountability. 'Working collectively' could be seen as a safe way for an organisation to be radical in identity, up to a point, without rocking the boat too much. It can also obscure real differences of interest within a work group in not very helpful ways.

The obscuring of differences and a slowness in acknowledging change are both features of group life at the Women's Therapy Centre. This reluctance to acknowledge change is probably a characteristic of *all* groups, but an unwillingness to admit difference seems to be especially pronounced in an all-women's group. A reason for this proposed by object-relations theorists such as Isabel Menzies and Elliot Jaques, is that groups function for their members as mechanisms of defence against powerful fears and anxieties of a primitive kind to do with separation and dependency. Any kind of individual differentiation threatens these group defence mechanisms and is usually, therefore, strongly resisted by the group. That would be the end of it and no change in groups would ever occur, were it not for the fact that each individual in a group is also deeply and inescapably committed to her own individual development and getting her own (individual) needs met. The situation in groups is therefore in a state of dynamic tension, varying between being a collection of differentiated adults working together co-operatively to achieve common goals, and being a collection of group members unconsciously driven to preserve their collective defences against the nameless fears aroused by the 'questioning attitude'. Bion, in *Experiences in Groups*, named these two types of group, respectively, the work group and the 'basic assumption' group. The work group he characterised as working at a conscious, rational level, drawing up goals and tasks and using its knowledge and skills to achieve them (not without difficulty and conflict). The 'basic assumption' group, on the other hand, seemed to act spontaneously and instinctively as though on the basis of some common emotional assumption, usually behind a leader, avoiding any reference to the demands of external reality as much as possible. Bion observed that groups fluctuated continually between being work groups and basic assumption groups. He divided the basic assumption group into three categories or types: the 'dependency', the 'fight-flight' and the 'pairing' group. Descriptions of these three types are given below for the benefit of the reader not acquainted with Bion's work on groups. They are offered as conceptual tools which may help to expose some of the muddles which occur in groups, and therefore begin to achieve some of the objectivity needed for the process of sorting them out.

The 'dependency' group acts as though it meets in order to be sustained by a leader (whether a person or an idea) on whom it depends for nourishment and protection. The group members act as though under the assumption that they themselves are inadequate, empty and immature, whereas the leader is omniscient and omnipotent. No investigation of this belief in the leader is allowed until such time as her idealisation can no longer be sustained, at which time she is rapidly devalued and replaced by another. There is a constant, vague feeling of frustration in the group at being unable to extract as much knowledge, goodness and power from the leader as is desired, and at the outside world, which is experienced as empty and disappointing.

The 'fight-flight' group is a group mobilised for uncompromising fight or flight alone. The accepted leader is one whose demands on the group afford it the opportunity for flight or aggression only. All other demands, for example, for analysis or development, will be ignored. Any opposition to the 'ideology' shared by the majority of the group cannot be tolerated, and the group easily splits into sub-groups which fight each other. Frequently, one sub-group is subservient to the idealised leader, while another sub-group attacks or is in flight from it. Suspicion, aggression and fear are the dominant emotions.

The 'pairing' group focuses on two of its members, a couple, who symbolise the group's hopeful expectation that through them it will be regenerated and preserved. The group is suffused with feelings of anticipation, even excitement, at the prospect of the, as yet unborn, new idea, person or project which will resolve all its difficulties. There can be feelings of shared intimacy within the group, almost sexual in nature, which serve as a protection against feelings of dependency and aggression.

Bion's categories can be helpful in discerning whether a group is actually behaving as rationally as it claims in pursuing its overt goals, or whether it is in the grip of one of the basic emotional assumptions, and therefore unlikely to be effective, or amenable to rational argument. The relationship between the group and its leader of the moment is usually a clue as to which type of group has the ascendancy. In the work group, leadership is functional: whoever has the necessary knowledge, experience and skills for the task takes the lead. No such qualifications are required of the basic assumption group leader, who can have the enthusiastic allegiance of the group but be devoid of any contact with reality other than the reality of the basic assumption group's demands, which are that she be a 'magician' or behave like one, giving an illusion of security. There is little overt disagreement with a basic assumption group leader, although she may be replaced if she fails to live up to the group's idealisations or meet their unconscious demands.

Before having read any of Bion's work, I had been aware for some time of a phenomenon of group life at the Women's Therapy Centre which is probably common to most small work groups: that there were some women within the group whose pronouncements were almost never questioned or challenged. I noticed this because, often, although I would have liked to question some of the points they made myself, I felt unable to do so because it seemed far too dangerous an undertaking. It was as though they were the custodians of the group's 'feminist' identity in some way, and to question them was a threat, either to this identity, or to my own eligibility to be a group member. Not everyone occupied this unchallengeable position. Clearly there were some people within the group with whom it was much safer to disagree. So it wasn't as though the phenomenon could be entirely explained by our individual difficulties in handling conflict, although of course these exist. It was more that we experienced those difficulties consistently in relation to some group members rather than to others. I have found it helpful to be aware that the WTC group, like any other group, behaves at times like a basic assumption group in this way.

A women's organisation that pins its identity on being 'feminist' is probably specially prone to behave as a basic assumption group at times, particularly once the original leaders who gave the group that definition have left. Though physically absent, the group may use them, or those they see as closest to them, as the leaders of a 'dependency' group. Similarly, the idea that there exists an organisational structure that is inherently 'feminist' may also become the leader of a 'dependency' group. Even to question this idea, as this article has begun to do, may *feel* like threatening the group with extinction. Similarly, to propose that the Centre consult more with outside groups and let them in to the policy-making process may arouse a 'fight-flight' defence, as though 'they' will stop us in some way from being a 'feminist' group. Perhaps, as Menzies suggests, these anxieties are a defence against the fear of internal changes taking place within individuals in relation to their feminist beliefs, or about our own dependency needs, particularly in relation to the 'male' world. A third defence can be that the group puts all its hope for the future into a 'pair' within the group whose combined creative powers will be able to produce a solution to its problems, whether through a massive private fund-raising drive, for example, or an educational programme which will convert a hostile world and guarantee the future.

All this is *not* to argue that the real financial and political difficulties faced by most women's organisations at present are the result merely of the group's own pathology. Neither is it to argue that an increased understanding of group dynamics will save us all. (To believe so would be, itself, to fall victim to one of the basic assumptions.) Some group analytic concepts can, though, offer insights and help in daring to ask questions and rethink some of our most dearly held assumptions about what we mean by working according to feminist or radical principles.

> The first requirement for effective functioning of an organiz-ation – including its leadership – is the adequate relationship between the organization's overall task and its administrative structure; the task has to be meaningful rather than trivial and, given the available resources, feasible rather than over-whelming.[9]

When these requirements are not met, the task group structure breaks down and the group processes within the organisation regress in the way that Bion has described. And we regress for good reasons: defining our aims, assessing whether they are feasible and whether we have the resources to achieve them, taking a cool look at our administrative structure, are all immensely difficult tasks. They are not just consciously diffi-cult, they can also arouse unconscious terrors of aggression and annihilation, the converse of our longing to be merged with the group, like an infant with its mother.

Carole Sturdy

Acknowledgment

I would like to thank Jean Thomson and all the women at the Women's Therapy Centre for their encouragement and support in writing this article.

Notes

1.   Wilfred Bion, *Experiences in Groups*, Tavistock Publications, London, 1961, p.162.
2.   Isabel Menzies, 'The function of social systems as a defence against anxiety: a report on a study of the nursing service of a general hospital', *Tavistock Pamphlet no. 3,* Tavistock Institute of Human Relations, London, 1970; Elliott Jaques, 'Social systems as defence against persecutory and depressive anxiety', in M. Klein, P. Heimann, and R. Money-Kyrle, *New Directions in Psychoanalysis*, Maresfield Library, London 1985; and Otto F. Kernberg. 'Leadership and organisational functioning' in *International Journal of Group Psychotherapy*, New York, 1978, Volume 28.
3.   Sheila Rowbotham, Lynne Segal and Hilary Wainwright, *Beyond the Fragments*, Merlin Press, London, 1979, p.30.
4.   Charles Landry, David Morley, Russell Southwood and Patrick Wright, *What a Way to Run a Railroad*, Comedia Publishing Group, London, 1985, p.13.
5.   Charles Handy, *Understanding Organizations*, Penguin, Harmondsworth, 1976, p.210.
6.   Charles Handy, 'Volorgs', in *MDU Bulletin*, Management Development Unit at NCVO, No. 5, June 1985.
7.   Landry *et al.*, *What a Way to Run a Railroad*, p.49.
8.   Charles Handy, *Understanding Organizations*, p.185.
9.   Otto F. Kernberg, 'Leadership and organisational functioning' p.4.

3
Separation and intimacy: crucial practice issues in working with women in therapy

The question is often posed: What is different about feminist therapy? Murmurings ensue and some examples are given. 'Oh', the unimpressed questioner retorts, 'but that would happen in any "good therapy." The respondent works hard to bring up more examples, to show the basis from which interventions are made, to insist on the differences, to describe the atmosphere in the therapy relationship, to discuss 'feminist' understandings of transference and countertransference and so on. The dialogue tends to be unsatisfactory. The questioner may be looking to prove that there are political/propagandist elements: the respondent may feel under pressure to define feminist therapy in relation to other psychotherapies rather than in terms of itself. The discussion thus proceeds on a disagreeable basis. The questioner and the respondent miss each other, they are not talking the same language.[1]

This mismatching is not accidental. It reflects the antagonism that has greeted feminist psychotherapy. Since feminist psychotherapy makes no pretence to be non-political (as opposed to other therapies which claim to be value-free, objective or simply interested in the individual) one might surmise that the anger is directed at the political nature of the therapy. To a certain extent this is the case. Psychoanalysis, humanistic psychology, transactional analysis, phenomenology, existential psychotherapy, gestalt psychotherapy and psychosynthesis, loudly declaim their political indifference and lack of bias. They rarely concede that their discipline, like feminist psychotherapy, expresses a particular world view.

However if the antagonism is not wholly engendered by the explicitly political level, where does it come from? We think it stems from the implications of the feminist position, i.e. what feminism tells us about women's requirements in therapy, and what an investigation of women's psychology reveals about the many devastatingly painful aspects of women's inner experience. Encountering these aspects of women's lives within the therapy relationship is difficult for the therapist. Since feminist therapy is relatively new, very few therapists working today have had the experience of undergoing feminist analysis themselves. It may well be the case that what they are required to do in their professional capacity is to provide a therapy relationship they themselves still wish to experience. Being able to foster and accept the expression of a great deal of pain from the client and, as we shall see, receiving this pain within aspects of the therapy relationship itself, can be extremely emotionally demanding. In addition, what comes up for the client inevitably speaks to issues in the therapist's life forcing a continual recognition of the shared nature of women's oppression.

Feminist investigations in psychoanalysis have exposed the serious consequences of patriarchy. These are insights people are inclined to feel extremely uncomfortable about for two main reasons. Firstly, these insights have implications for the conduct of the therapy itself. The therapeutic relationship is transformed by a feminist understanding and intention. Feminist therapy does not simply 'tack on' women's issues to therapeutic practice. As we shall see it profoundly affects the structure and the understanding of the therapeutic dialogue. It reframes the terms of the therapy relationship. Secondly, it becomes obvious that even a personal solution cannot be found simply within the therapeutic practice.[2] An interpretation that speaks to the full meaning of an individual woman's experience reflects an understanding of the ways in which the material world creates individual personality, symptomatology, defence structures and so on. Out of this it becomes clear that nothing short of a restructuring of social arrangements is required if the conditions that give rise to women's present psychological position are to change fundamentally.

Feminist therapy takes as its starting point that women have a social existence and that femininity (women's psychology) is formed within a particular social context. Society is not a collection of individuals, as in the Freudian view, but is rather what makes and defines individual human possibilities. Thus psychologies always reflect in complex ways prevailing social mores. In our society these mores lay a stress on the individual notion of the self – a self raised within a patriarchal nuclear family. The most critical features of a girl's development to womanhood depend upon the relationships and social institutions that interact with her developing self. Mothering is thus not simply an individual relationship, it is a social institution. Fathering is not simply an individual relationship, it is a social institution. What takes place in mothering and fathering is extremely complex but it is always reflective of the social laws of patriarchy. The relating that occurs, the feelings that are generated, the obligations rendered and sought, the fantasies and longings, are psychological indicators of what is possible and what is not possible within the current social order.

What feminist psychotherapy at the theoretical level tries to uncover is the structure that governs familial relations so that the process towards femininity can be better understood. What it tries to do at the clinical level is take account of the impact of these structures on the developing psyche. What the psychotherapy attempts to achieve (i.e. in conventional terms what would constitute a 'cure') is not so much a coming to terms with these structures – as in classical analysis where the acceptance of the oedipal resolution is considered evidence of a successful analysis – but a grappling with the implications of these structures so that the effects can be challenged. This is an important idea and a foundation stone of feminist psychotherapy – which is concerned with not simply identifying the structures that psychically make us who we are but with psychic restructuring so that the very parameters of femininity (and masculinity) are expanded and changed. Feminist therapy has revealed depths of suffering that exist for many many women. Consequently, just as feminism fights on the political front to restructure public life, feminist psychotherapy focuses on the individual psyche and the restructuring in the here and now of aspects of private life. What then are the hallmarks of femininity as we presently know it and experience it? What are the psychological costs, the ramifications of socialisation to the feminine role? And what are the psychological equivalents and effects of women's public subordination?

A woman's psychology is defined to a very large extent by her designated social role as mother. This is true whether or not she takes up the (very recent) option to be a mother. The structure of parenting in which women mother is almost universal within the Western world, and thus appears natural, but in exploring developmental psychology we can see the psychological imperatives that structure this role and the ways in which mothering occurs. We can see *how* a girl comes to be a mothering person and we can discern the shape which that gives to her psyche. When we are looking at a woman, we are looking at the psychology of someone who has, in some measure or another, been brought up to take on the social role of caregiver and nurturer, to introduce infants and children to appropriate ways of feeling and behaving, to be the provider of the continuity between generations, the person responsible for the continuity in relating, and so on.

Mothering then, not mothering in the biological sense of the capacity to give birth, but in the sense of the socially established notions of what goes along with being a mothering person, is a key feature of femininity. When women break away from these aspects of their personality or when they feel inadequate with established practices as givers and nurturers they suffer dis-ease. Little girls are brought up to be women who will have an awareness of the needs of others, who will minister to those needs – even to anticipate them before their articulation and demonstration. Women come to provide comfort and emotional support services to those around them: family, co-workers, bosses. Operationally, this means that much of a woman's energy is directed to working out what others desire so that she may respond appropriately. Frequently it will require that she defer to those desires.

A second determining feature of woman's social role – again the notional norm until very recently – is linked with the idea that a woman has only reached adulthood and been 'successful' as a woman when she has connected herself with a man. This connection is conceived of as important and yet highly difficult to achieve, so that in order to secure a man (or maybe we should say 'get one' – securing is something else altogether!) she must make herself into someone that others will find appealing. When she finds her man, her social status and how she is perceived in the world still largely depend upon his location in society. Adult separate womanhood is not a category that has until this last decade received any open respect or legitimation.

These two determining features of a woman's social role – being a mother and getting a man – have a profound effect on her psychology. They shape it in particular ways and are instrumental in creating certain kinds of feelings she has about herself. They operate in the most obvious and in the most subtle and unconscious ways. Let's take the most obvious first and then we will sketch some of the developmental steps that ensue in the process towards femininity.

The conceiving of oneself as a nurturing, mothering type of person, who responds to the desires of others and defers to them, has what can be considered both negative and positive consequences for the woman's psychology. To start with what feminist psychologists, Jean Baker Miller[3] and Carol Gilligan[4] have seen as positive, the capacity to relate to others, to care for them and to think about them, creates a way of being that is people-orientated rather than instrumental. At first glance it is a version of the 'being' state that Winnicott[5] refers to. Feminine emotional values of care, concern and outerdirectedness are represented as important rather than the values of competition, success in the world, and so on. That these values are not socially validated should not lead us to reject them, Jean Baker Miller suggests, for they are the skills that although acquired through women's location as subordinate, are nevertheless positive and represent a bulwark against the damaging values our public culture stands for.

This position seems to us valid up to a point. It is important to legitimate feminine values and feminine morality and to cast women's psychological development in its own terms rather than in inevitable contrast to male psychology. However, the obvious negative consequences of this way of being revolve around the creation of a personality which, needing to be on the alert all the time to respond to others, has little chance to develop its own needs. Moreover, and this is our general problem with this positive view, it would seem to elevate a consequence of oppression into a virtue. While undoubtedly it is a good thing that we have developed these skills of caring, they have complex implications that need to be addressed. Far from achieving the 'being' state, the demands of giving, frequently built on a base of deprivation, render women continually psychically busy so that they are chronically in the Winnicottian 'doing' rather than 'being' state. Further, the conception that one's own needs are important and worthy of being addressed by oneself or by others, is missing. The self is validated in emotional service rather than through being directly related to. Many women express their response to this state of affairs in the everyday language of feeling, saying that something is missing, that they do not quite know who they are or what they want, or they may say that when they are in a close relationship they 'lose' themselves, or that when a relationship ends they no longer know who they are.

Let's turn briefly to what women in therapy present, for there can be no more dramatic exposure of this tragic underbelly than the painful states women reveal in the consulting room.[6] Listening to women who come to therapy, there is a remarkable similarity in the content of what they say and the way in which they perceive themselves. Of course in the therapy relationship, particularly in the beginning, the things women share about themselves tend to be in the areas of dissatisfaction. Nevertheless it is startling to realise quite how low women's self-esteem is. Women remark frequently on how basically at fault they are or how inadequate they are in essential ways. They feel that there is a disjuncture between the way they show themselves and are seen to be adults in the world, and their internal experience of insecurity and uncertainty. They worry that if people could see through them they would discover the frequently frightened, nervous and angry little girl inside who is not at all sure where she does belong in relation to others.[7]

Women talk of the consequences of seeking self-definition through relating to others. The relating becomes so enmeshed that they have a difficult time experiencing their own identity as a separate free-standing person who relates with other separate people. Women talk of how they stay in unsatisfactory relationships fearing a loss of self if they were to withdraw from the relationship. They seek new relationships, driven by the need not simply for connection but for identity.

This need for connection is linked with the social requirements of feminine deference and submission. Women discuss how habitual deference to others militates against developing their own opinions. Women encourage others to express their wants and ideas and then use those as reference points for their own thoughts and feelings. When a woman does express an opinion, she may be preoccupied with the reactions of others. Under such circumstances, dissent or conflict often induces a kind of panic. Controversy is experienced not simply as difference but as potentially dangerous, and for some it is felt as a sort of annihilating differentiation. Of course, in therapy, as in consciousness-raising groups where women first gave vent to their feelings in a self-conscious way, it becomes obvious that when given the opportunity of being listened to, women have many strong opinions and clear thoughts about most situations they find themselves in. Their deference and lack of confidence does not accurately reflect their lack of thought or opinion but rather their socially derived psychological position.

Women in therapy discuss how complicated the emotion of anger can be. It is a feeling that can cause great difficulty. It can be experienced as uncomfortable and even dangerous for it goes against the grain. It is an assertion of one's self in relation to another, an act of differentiation. As such it is somewhat incompatible with notions of the primacy of others' experience. Women's unease with acknowledging or expressing their anger creates a situation in which they fear that it is enormously powerful. They fear it could alienate at least, annihilate at most, the person towards whom it is directed. They fear they will lose what little they have.

In therapy, an internalised critical part of woman's psyche presents itself starkly. It is as though women carry around a third eye, a kind of punitive judge, who watches every action, thought and interaction closely. More often than not the judge finds fault. She has done something wrong or shown herself to be greedy in her needs and desires. The internal judge is keenly aware of the specific relational contexts in which women must live and constantly reminds her to be supremely aware of others' feelings. The judge assesses the effect she is having on another person and, depending upon whether she has been deferring and caretaking appropriately or inappropriately, engenders feelings of guilt, remorse or gratification.

Beyond such specifics, a common and critical feeling that so many women voice is that of a despairing hopelessness of ever being truly understood. Women rarely have the expectation that another person will be interested enough to really listen. To listen not in order to interpret, diagnose or offer ideas for change, but rather to listen in an attempt to understand and make contact with all aspects of who she is. Her inner life is confusing, painful and at times overwhelming. The idea that another woman could attentively engage with her is both frightening and exhilarating. It feels as though for so long, perhaps for as long as she can remember, she has always had to take care of herself and not to look to others for emotional understanding or nurturance. This has been so much of her way of being that finding herself on the receiving (rather than the active giving) end of a relationship in therapy can feel quite awkward, perplexing and poignant. It stirs up all kinds of needs, desires and longings which she has contained.

The question then arises of how women come so uniformly to have this kind of psychology – a psychology that means we frequently do not feel whole, we feel undeserving, and fraudulent in significant ways, we feel exhausted with all the giving that comes of being the emotional antennae, we feel that our real selves have either not emerged or if they were to do so they would be unattractive, and so on.

One of the advances that feminism has made possible has been to see the importance of mothers in the lives of women and in the forming of a woman's identity. (This focus has by no means been confined to psychology.[8]) Feminist scholarship in psychoanalysis[9] and other therapeutic disciplines has shed light on the structure of this relationship and it details the immense impact that the mother–daughter relationship has on feminine psychology. In doing so it has shifted the focus from the mother–son and father–daughter constellations, 'privileging' the mother–daughter relationship. In this relationship the mother, who has been raised as a woman herself, is the child's first most consistent and visible representative of the feminine. Who she is, how she is, how she feels about herself and what she projects about herself, powerfully inform the daughter's emotional and physical experiences of femininity and of mothering. They will influence how she feels about her mother and how she feels and conceives of femininity and mothering *for herself*. Beyond this obvious but often neglected reality are the many dynamics in the mother–daughter relationship, dynamics that occur as a result of this relationship shouldering the burden of the social and psychological requirements necessary for the reproduction of femininity.

Before we go into some of the specifics it is important to remind ourselves of the social context in which this relating occurs and the imperatives that attach to it. The mother is placed in a problematic position. An important part of mothering involves providing an environment in which her children can come to take up their designated masculine and feminine roles. She is instrumentally engaged in the process by which the sexed neonate becomes a gendered person. In other words, it rests upon her (or the primary caretaker, who tends to be a mother substitute and therefore for the purposes of this argument we shall refer to as the mother) to bring to life the psychological birth[10] of her infant. A most important feature of that psychological birth – the experiencing of oneself as a subject in relation to other subjects – is the perception of oneself as a male or as a female subject.

Gender is inextricable from our notions of subjectivity. The ordering of the sexes is a fundamental characteristic of human development. In enabling her infants to assume a gendered sense of self, the mother relates to them in gender-appropriate ways. This occurs on two different levels simultaneously. One is in regard to appropriate sex-role stereotyping; the other in shaping their psychological sense of self. In the first of these, she introduces a boy to the ways that her world deems appropriate to being a boy and she introduces a girl to the suitable ways of being a girl. This means that she relates differentially to them, encouraging different aspects of their personalities so that they will broadly conform to the sex-role stereotypes of their culture. While it might be protested that mothers do not do anything so crude as sex-typing their children, one would be hard put to find many mothers who are comfortable with their boys wearing pretty dresses (except in a dressing-up game) or many who are at ease with their girls playing with toy automatic rifles. At a less obvious level we can notice how boys are routinely encouraged to confront and overcome the implicit dangers in an adventure playground. A mother may grit her teeth and bear it as she watches him career through some treacherous pole vault. She may find it far more of a challenge to contain her anxiety when a daughter wishes to do the same thing. She may indicate that the danger is one to be avoided, not one to be mastered (*sic*). What we all *feel* as opposed to *think* about what boys and girls can/should do is deeply influenced by cultural prescriptions in the most explicit and the most subtle of ways.[11]

The simultaneous but more subtle, and frequently unconscious, ways in which the mother–daughter relationship guides our taking up our gendered positions is of principal concern to us in coming to grips with understanding women's inner experience. The way in which the mothering person presents the psychological possibilities that exist are shaped by many factors. They include the mother's own experience of being mothered, they rest on her conscious and unconscious feelings about having a daughter, her identification with a same-sexed child, and they are influenced by the kind of support she receives in parenting, and her own internal object relations. All of these factors are framed within the social matrix of the mother, who as a member of the subordinate sex is charged with bringing up her daughter to assume a similar social position. This is the problematic of the mother–daughter relationship.

The relationship is set within excruciating parameters. The oppressed mother must negotiate her relationship with her daughter around and within the fact of her own subordination. She may well wish to transform the possibilities that exist for her daughter and encourage her to break free of some of the confines of femininity. She may on the other hand, be uncritical of her own position or upbringing, seeking to provide mothering and guidelines for life on the lines that she herself experienced. Most commonly, mothering includes a mixture of contradictory conscious and unconscious stances which express a playing out of the various possibilities in relation to women's social subordination. But however the subtle variations play out in each mother—daughter relationship, that relationship is nevertheless constrained by wider social practices. It is an ironic and cruel phenomenon of patriarchy that the already oppressed shall prepare the succeeding generation for a similar fate.

Fundamental to the uptake of femininity is the taboo on dependency and the taboo on initiating.[12] That is to say, her actions, large and small, which proclaim her own existence, and attempt to define her boundaries and are constrained by the responses she receives. Girls are brought up to provide a supportive relationship and an emotional lifeline for others. In this context they learn to service the needs of others and come to identify the satisfaction of *their* needs with the meeting of those needs in others. This overarching dictate is conveyed by the mother to the daughter in distinct ways. On the one hand, the daughter is encouraged to play co-operatively, to be a little mother, to pay attention to other children's wants, to be kind and solicitous. These personality characteristics are praised and encouraged. At the same time, it is indicated to the daughter that she should develop the facility to contain her own neediness. She grows up without the expectation that her emotional needs will be attended to. This dictate finds expression in the mother—daughter relationship itself. The mother, unnurtured herself and weary from all the giving out that she is doing, frequently looks to her daughter to be especially solicitous to her. In teaching her to be thoughtful and caring towards others she herself becomes a candidate for such attention from her daughter. A cycle in which 'giving' occurs out of unmet personal needs is thus set in train. The mother becomes the daughter's first child.

This stress on giving and attending to the needs of others inevitably thwarts the daughter's development towards differentiation and autonomy. Awareness of the other is ever present. She initiates within the context of behaviours that are sanctioned. She restricts initiatives on behalf of self which seem to threaten connection in relationships. Gradually she loses the facility to clearly identify needs and desires that arise internally. Such needs become a manifestation of what is possible. Needs that are impermissible either do not surface or do so with hesitancy and fear. Eventually, desire *itself* is felt as precarious. Thus a girl's psychology develops with a fear and repression of her own needs and wishes. These unmet needs are consciously and unconsciously rejected by the girl who then comes to understand them, and consequently a part of herself, as bad. An illegitimacy, a sense of undeserving and unentitlement follow. As she grows up her psychology embodies feelings of unworthiness and self-hate.

Now we have drawn a picture of women's psychology it is possible briefly to see how an orthodox and a feminist therapy in turn might view these same features and how they might go about responding to the woman's dilemma and the pain that is inevitably generated by socialisation to femininity.

We think it is no exaggeration to claim that orthodox psychotherapies tend to view women's problems as we have discussed them, as the manifestation of a truncated pre-oedipal development. In other words, the insecurity a woman may feel, the way she may inhibit her desires, her conflicts around dependency, come to be seen as expressions of her insatiability and her continuing need for the primary love object. She continues to hold on, making separation problematic. The course of treatment focuses on the ambivalence of separation. Although we are representing this position in rather a crude way it is undoubtedly the prevailing practice within psychoanalytic therapy. For example, it is hard to sit through a lecture or seminar or a supervisory session in which a woman client is being discussed without hearing the shorthand phrases such as 'she needs to separate', 'she hasn't separated yet'. The implication being that it is the therapist's task to focus the work in the direction of separation. Indeed many a therapist has been heard to remark, 'The process of separation is one that starts in the first session and continues through to the last.' In this approach, separation from the mother is the *sine qua non* of the therapeutic endeavour. The patient/client must come to accept that she cannot get what she needs from her mother. She should work through (i.e. give up) the longing and accept the loss of what she cannot have. Having done so, and 'separated' she will be in a position to take what a heterosexual relationship in the present can offer.

While on the face of it this is an eminently sensible proposition (of course she cannot get now what she did not get then from her mother), the pursuit of such a course too uncomfortably reflects the social realities of women's subordination, which are that she should not expect continued nurturance, that she should accept her lot, that she should resolve not to want. It is isomorphic with women's daily experience. It implies that her wanting is over-abundant and must be curtailed. If she can come to grips with wanting less then she will be able to partake of what is there for her.

With this diagnosis and the therapeutic effort being expended towards separation, the therapeutic work proceeds towards a restructuring of the defence structure. An attempt to relate to the unmet/unseparated self is abandoned in favour of a thrust to stabilise it more firmly behind a defence structure. The proposed forms of the separation contribute, we fear, to a consolidation of a Winnicottian 'false self'. The woman learns to inhibit her needs more effectively. As a result she may well feel temporarily less out of control, or less in danger of being overwhelmed by them but, in essence, psychic change has been directed towards a *change in the defence structure* rather than resolving the discrepancy between the embryonic undeveloped self and the defences. The therapist and client come to collude in a process in which the woman client's needs are once again de-legitimised. A shared assumption is that the need is something one must negotiate rather than see if it can be met. (It is a non-struggle position for the therapist, an indication of *her* hopelessness that women can receive and digest the emotional nurturance they so evidently require.) A parallel that might make this clearer is the idea that a compulsive eater will solve her food problems through dieting. Such a response is not a solution *per se*. A diet is but a short-term measure to hold back the desire towards food by channelling it in a particular direction. The 'compulsivity' manifest in the distressed eating behaviour is now harnessed to obsessive practices about what one should and shouldn't eat. The desire is held back rather than addressed, investigated and met.

Such an approach seems oddly atherapeutic until one considers the political background to psychotherapeutic thinking. For putting the stress on separation is rather like blaming the victim. The woman is condemned for what she has not had. (Poor people are blamed for their poverty.) Women always strive to get what they need, often in circuitous or indirect ways. It is an expression of strength and the urgency of their unmet needs that alerts women to being such good caregivers to others. It is the indirect expression and the systematic transposition into giving to others that causes women such tremendous stress. For the feminist psychotherapist then, we can see that the issue is surely not one in which she is implicitly encouraging the client/patient to give up the wanting, nor for her to accept the expectation of not getting. What is required rather is that a woman receive encouragement to struggle for what she needs, to have that wanting accepted as legitimate and understandable. In other words, the woman's desire needs to be recognised now and looked at straightforwardly rather than pushed underground once again.

In so far as it is manifest as a present wanting for authentic relating, then this desire needs to be *and can be* met in the therapeutic relationship. The task of feminist therapy is to address the original not-getting and to provide an experience of consistent caring that can be ingested in the present. Of course this does not imply that the therapist can 'make up' for the loss the woman carries with her. However the present contact can carry the sorrow, rage, upset and confusion surrounding past unmet need while meeeting the need for relating that occurs in the present. As we shall see, it is the working through the defences *against* such a kind of relating that forms a central focus of the therapeutic work.

Perhaps now we are getting to one of the crucial differences between a feminist approach and other approaches. The feminist approach accepts, indeed anticipates, that the mother–daughter relationship is bound to be ambivalent and problematic and that its legacy is that the daughter (and indeed the mother herself as a daughter) is unable to separate. However it does not view or define this problem in the same terms as those of the other approaches. Nor does it view the woman's developmental schema in terms of pre-oedipal and oedipal stages with the latter constituting the greater achievement. Rather it views the vicissitudes of the mother–daughter relationship in its own terms, and sees its impact on the course of the other relationships with which the daughter engages. In 'privileging' this relationship, it speaks to the problematic that is posed by the mother–daughter relationship. It speaks to the issues not in separation *per se* but to the difficulties that have occurred in the original merger and the subsequent impact these have on the achievement of *intimacy and connection*.

Separation, we contend, is such a very difficult area for women because it rests on the dilemma of the person who has not yet had sufficient emotional supplies to consolidate a psychological sense of self which can allow for a genuine separation. In other words, from our perspective, it is not separation that is fundamentally at issue, it is intimacy. At first glance it might appear that women are fluent in the area of emotional intimacy – and indeed such a claim has great force when set against men's general ineptitude in this area. Women do know how to get close to one another, they do know that intimacy is something they seek and value, they do routinely engage in encounters that reflect some intimacy. However, that much desired intimacy brings its own set of problems. In intimate relating there is a rapidity in the dissolution of boundaries between self and other. This dissolution and the resultant psychological merger with another may be greatly desired and/or may be met with great trepidation. A temporary psychological merger with another is especially precarious if one is unsure of the boundaries of the self in the first place. The merger is much wished for but may be felt to be dangerous for one may feel stuck in it. The falsely constructed boundaries between self and other so endemic in women's psychology hide an undeveloped and shaky sense of self identity. The merger may feel like a 'loss of whatever sense of self' one has garnered. (Thus women will often say 'I know who I am when I am not in a relationship, but I lose myself when I am in love.') Beyond this loss, intimate relating, in providing a feeling, however brief, of being understood and met, can be excruciating for it can stir up all the longing that has for so long gone unmet and hence has been repressed and denied.

In the therapy relationship the defence structure and the defences that are manifest are most profoundly defences against intimacy. Intimacy with the therapist is the most wanted and yet the most feared event. Intimacy experienced with the therapist is felt to be so painful that almost before it has been digested it gets undone, or there is a retreat from it. One can observe this within the flow of an individual session and over the course of several sessions. The desire for contact is so profound and so unknown that steps towards disengagement and towards what might appear to be separation are rife. The client's assertion that she does not need any more after just a few sessions or later on that she is doing better and could stop therapy now, have significance in this context. They are frequently the utterances of the defence against intimacy. They are not signposts towards a genuine separation. For this reason, the work we do focuses much attention on the minutiae of movement and nuance *within* the therapy relationship: the impact of the contact between the client and therapist; its implications and how it can be used as the nourishment for the development of the client's embryonic self; the lack of trust that such contact can be relied upon; the playing over time and again of the same worry that the client feels herself to be too needy and too burdensome; the retreats from the contact (by client and by the therapist) and the ways in which these are understood and worked through in the therapeutic dyad.

Out of such an examination comes a different kind of contact, one that is less staccato than the original push—pull of the mother—daughter relationship.[13] It is a contact that allows for the genuine development of a sense of self that permeates all of the woman so that she can engage with others without the concomitant loss of self (which occurs when a shaky defence structure is pierced, rendering an undeveloped self vulnerable) or the compromise of not getting. In this way both the taboo against the meeting of women's dependency needs and the taboo against initiating are challenged. The woman's needs that arise in the therapy relationship are acknowledged, as well as her fears of the exposure of those needs. In providing a complete interpretation (i.e. speaking to the need and to the defence) the therapist goes some way towards them being met. In the process of the needs being addressed the client is transformed. She no longer views herself as a needy person who must curb whatever comes up in her. She no longer feels herself to be unentitled and unworthy. She no longer suffers a gargantuan split between the private and the public. This begins to shift the motivational basis from which women's caretaking comes. It allows the woman to give and receive out of a wholeness rather than from the compelling need to attach out of an incomplete sense of self. Her hesitancy now in regard to the expression of her own desire reflects an engagement with social reality rather than with personal feelings of illegitimacy.

All this is not to say that a feminist orientated therapy as described can in any sense alleviate the inequities of the world. The world at large will not suddenly appear benevolent and available because the individual woman has been able to take in nourishment in therapy and build up a psychological self. The world may still be experienced as hostile and this will not be simply a projection. For the world *is* hostile to women. It discourages their initiatives, it denigrates their desires. It silences women in various explicit and subtle says. A feminist understanding in psychology does not change the outer world, but it may alter the woman's ability to cope with it. It will not provide for 'adjustment' to the social mores but it brings their relationship to the individual's psychology into sharp relief.

Susie Orbach and Luise Eichenbaum

Notes

1. A crucial aspect of feminist therapy is the finding of a language, a mode of communication that reverses the historical mismatching of the client's needs. Dale Spender and others looking at speech and language have pointed out how crucial language is in the formation of consciousness and access to power. The language of therapy is a language that speaks to an often hidden area of women's experience. It is not the language of everyday life, nor is it the language routinely used in discussions about women clients in settings which eschew a feminist input.

2. For Freud, a reasonable therapeutic goal was the transformation from neurosis to 'ordinary unhappiness'. We, on the other hand, anticipate that the individual woman will be able to live more fully and contentedly but that she will carry with her in addition the conscious knowledge and consequences of her social position and the various meanings that that can have in her personal relationships. It is in this sense that we mean there is no such thing as a personal solution. One cannot exclude women's oppression from one's awareness. It is a feature of our lives and of how our personalities have been constructed that we wrestle with continually..

3. Jean Baker Miller, *Towards a New Psychology of Women*, Penguin, Harmondsworth, 1978.

4. Carol Gilligan, *In a Different Voice*, Harvard University Press, Cambridge, Mass., 1982.

5. D.W. Winnicott, *The Maturational Processes and the Facilitating Environment*, Hogarth Press, London, 1965.

6. This is not to say that this underbelly only affects women in therapy. Psychoanalysis has always taken as legitimate the generation of theory from the in-depth analysis of individual cases, seeing them as on the continuum of personality development.

7. This operates on both a conscious and unconscious level.

8. See for example Nancy Friday, *My Mother My Self*, New York, 1978; Judith Arcana, *Our Mother's Daughters*, The Women's Press, London, 1979; Adrienne Rich, *Of Woman Born: motherhood as experience and institution*, Virago, London, 1977; Elena Giannini Belotti, *Little Girls*, Writers and Readers, London, 1977.

9. Nancy Chodorow, *The Reproduction of Mothering: psychoanalysis and the sociology of gender*, University of California Press, Berkeley, Cal., 1978.
10. Margaret S. Mahler, Fred Pine and Anni Bergman, *The Psychological Birth of the Human Infant*, Basic Books, New York, 1975.
11. John Money and Anke Erhardt, *Man and Woman, Boy and Girl: the differentiation and dimophism of gender identity from conception to maturity*, John Hopkins University Press, Baltimore, Md., 1973.
12. Luise Eichenbaum and Susie Orbach, *What Do Women Want? exploding the myth of dependency*, Michael Joseph, London, 1983.
13. Luise Eichenbaum and Susie Orbach, *Understanding Women: a feminist psychoanalytic approach*, Basic Books, New York, 1982.

4
Can a daughter be a woman?
Women's identity and psychological separation

Freud neglected to ask how a woman comes into possession of her own story, becomes a subject, when even narrative convention assigns her the place of an object of desire. How does an object tell a story?[1]

Introduction

As feminists we have long recognised the ways in which patriarchal society has blocked women from having socially recognised and valued identities. A large part of our struggle has been directed towards gaining this social recognition and the economic and political changes it necessitates. The starting point of our struggle has been the establishment of an autonomous women's movement.

As a psychotherapist and a feminist I am also concerned with the relationship between women's external devaluation and lack of power and the individual woman's personal experience of lack of identity, of not being the subject of her own story. The source of this experience, I suggest, lies in the particular nature of the unconscious process of psychological separation of daughter from mother during early childhood; a process which is affected at each phase by the social experience of womanhood. Throughout the paper the emphasis is on the complexity of the interrelationship between social and psychological levels and the need for detailed study to elucidate the connections.

The terms personal identity and psychological separation are often used as if they were interchangeable, defined in Rycroft's *Dictionary of Psychoanalysis* as, 'The sense of one's continuous being as an entity distinguishable from all others'.[2] As Rycroft points out this definition covers both the subjective sense of one's existence and purpose in the world (whether conscious or unconscious) which I shall call 'identity' and the unconscious process 'by which the infant achieves mental detachment from the mother, that is, differentiation into a separate personal self',[3] which I shall refer to as separation. A daughter who is apparently autonomous in directing her own life, having a clear sense of identity, may unconsciously be living her life according to her fantasies of how her mother would perceive her and cannot therefore be seen as psychologically separate.

I have found it illuminating to look at the development of women's political consciousness alongside psychoanalytic accounts of the separation/individuation process. I am struck by the parallels between the two accounts and also by the inter-relationship between them: the difficulties that girls have in establishing their psychological separateness are affected by growing up in a culture in which only certain aspects of their femaleness are recognised. It is in the very essence of women's politics that we should be concerned with understanding the formation of the female psyche. There are accounts of children reared by wolves, or in total isolation, who do not develop the usual human capacities because their first burblings and movements are not reflected back appropriately or encouraged within their own environment. The experience for women is similar; certain aspects of ourselves are either not reflected back or are distorted so that we do not acquire the means of recognising or expressing those parts.

Describing women in the initial phase of women's revolutionary politics, Sheila Rowbotham wrote, 'We are like babes thrashing around in darkness and unexplored space.'[4] We need to be able to see ourselves, but, as she points out, the existing versions of femininity in a patriarchal society may only provide distorting mirrors. So we have to find or create mirrors which reflect ourselves more fully. She suggests that the first step we take towards this is to 'connect and learn to trust one another'.[5] In doing this a silence is broken, and we begin to hear and say things which we hardly knew we had experienced.

Marsha Rowe conveys some of the power and excitement of the early days of self-discovery in her description of the first meeting of women working in the underground press. 'The main impression that has stayed in my mind is of women voicing the other side of sexual permissiveness, talking of pain and anxiety about abortions – the discussion about work took second place to the one about sexuality. So much of our lives had been concealed from each other, it was as if we had been strangers. Other impressions were the way the room seemed to swirl with emotion so long suppressed and that I was frightened.'[6]

Women's discontent with their experience, whether it was housework, sexual permissiveness or how the doctor talked to them, had scarcely been articulated. There seemed to be a link between the apparent impossibility of changing things and the absence of words or concepts to articulate women's pain. When there is no hope of changing things there are no words or voices or concepts to express the need to change or the distress experienced. If the categories are available the pain becomes easier to recognise and acknowledge. 'The sound of silence breaking makes us understand what we could not hear before. But the fact that we could not hear does not prove that no pain existed.'[7]

Previously the hidden experiences had been conscious only in a sense of disjuncture between projected self-image and awareness of inner split or paralysis. 'We lumbered round ungainly-like in borrowed concepts which did not fit the shape we felt ourselves to be.'[8]

Beginning to recognise this, we had to return to our own experience, mirror it for each other, begin to construct our own visions of it, and to articulate these privately and publicly. The initial meeting that Marsha Rowe described was the forerunner of the women's liberation magazine *Spare Rib*. Sharing personal experience led to the production of a magazine in which many women could see their experiences described, analysed and reflected.

The concept of mirroring is a key one in much psychoanalytic writing on the earliest stages of infancy and is to be found in work of different theoretical orientations (for example, Winnicott, Lacan). It is used to describe a stage in the complex process whereby a child gains a sense of a world outside herself or himself and an image of her/his own existence within that world. Initially the child does not know where s/he ends and the world begins. There are many important parallels between these infantile processes and the difficulties women experience in achieving a sense of existing for themselves in the world. Studying the psychoanalytic work on the mirroring image Malcolm Pines writes of the 'self being actively mirrored by another responding self'.[9]

In Winnicott's account of infant development, which I shall look at in more detail later, he describes how the infant, needing to see herself* reflected literally in her mother's eyes and expression, begins to learn who s/he is. Inevitably the mother unconsciously selects what she reflects back. Mother and daughter's shared gender intensifies the mother's identification with her daughter.

Jane, who had had a particularly unsupportive relationship with her own mother, described her early response to her own first daughter: 'A persistent "I'm a bad mother" preoccupation began to swamp my pleasure in Kate . . . I heard her cries firstly as accusing me and only belatedly as a specific complaint to do with hunger, nappy rash, teething etc.'[10]

A mother who is feeling like this cannot *reflect back* the baby's expression of hunger, pain, anger or satisfaction. She is too encumbered by her daughter's re-evocation of her own early infancy. Unable to mirror the baby's feelings which the baby could 'recognise' as her own, the mother imposes her own feelings of being accused and persecuted on to the baby. Instead of having the experience of being safely mirrored by mother, the baby receives the unconscious message that these feelings are dangerous. The infant daughter may split off the

---

* I use 'herself' although Winnicott did not distinguish between the sexes in his work on early infancy. I shall use the term 'mother' for convenience but it should be understood to refer to the primary caretaker(s) whoever this may be.

aspects of herself which the mother has not been able to mirror. At the social level, continuing the metaphor of cultural reflection, many aspects of women's experience were never selected for reflection, prior to the women's movement. They too were hidden.

Those parts of the infant girl which are split off do not disappear but they are not available to be lived with in the growing child's imagination, expressed and tested out in relation to others and thus eventually integrated into the young child's psychic structure. In this way the toddler's tantrums eventually become the older child's outburst of anger when s/he feels wrongly treated by a friend or parent. Instead feelings which mother could not process are buried and thus maintain a power they would otherwise lose. The girl is left with a feeling that she lacks identity or a sense of self. In the outside world too the little girl's opportunities to experiment may be limited. Within the women's movement women found they needed to explore previously untouched dimensions of their inner worlds and to try out new ways of being as a preparation for the activities of organising, writing and creating new structures. Early women's groups often felt torn between consciousness-raising and political activity; now we can see the need for both. Once it was clear that women's oppression was inextricably linked with reproduction and the family, the need to articulate 'the delicate manner in which human beings stifle one another at the point of reproduction'[11] was acknowledged, as was the awareness that we would have to 'go back to the darkness of our unremembered childhood to understand the extent of our colonization'.[12] Having drawn parallels between women's cultural and psychological experience I suggest that while feminism creates a space within which women can begin to develop a social and cultural identity, so psychotherapy which incorporates this perspective can offer a similar space within which a woman can renegotiate her psychological separation. I also suggest that the separation process is an area of crucial interest for feminism because it illustrates the way in which we move into a relationship with the environment and how this is linked with the acquisition of gender identity.

The meaning of separation in some women's lives

'I used to feel like a drawing that anyone who wanted to could come along and rub out – there wasn't anything to me except my name and what I look like – I thought if only I can make a life for myself, a life like theirs, a life everyone would recognise as a life, then no-one could come along and rub me out.'[13]

Susan in Paul Scott's *The Jewel in the Crown* describes thus the subjective experience of not having a sense of self. This feeling of being a nobody which Susan talks of is an extreme form of an experience that many women may identify with. In the novels Susan's emptiness is explained at a social level in terms of the ending of the Raj and the way in which this revealed the true position of English women in India. In contrast, her sister Sarah understands the situation she is in, can look at it from the outside and bear with the painful perception of the absurdity of her life and that of her family. She is then able to find a role for herself within the inexorable movement towards the end of the Raj and the potential for a future outside colonial life.

Many of the heroines of feminist novels struggle, like Susan, to discover a sense of self and find this struggle most difficult when they are in an intimate relationship. Living in a different period from Susan many of these women *appear* to be leading independent lives with jobs or careers, but intimacy drags them right back into emotional subservience. In Sara Davidson's *Loose Change*[14] three of the Californian characters appear to be liberated; one is a successful journalist, another a rich art dealer and the third a much envied Berkeley radical having a relationship with a 'top' Berkeley student activist. Each in her own way loses her sense of self in a relationship with a man; none more so than Sue (the most overtly radical of the trio) who is even reduced to that old feminine trick – faking orgasms. Marge Piercy, too, has a series of heroines, such as Miriam in *Small Changes*[15] who appear vibrant to others (and even feel good themselves) but easily lose this and become clinging and desperate when they fall in love. Perhaps the prototype for this kind of heroine is Anna, the 'I' of Doris Lessing's *The Golden Notebook*,[16] who appears to have no control whatsoever over her relationships or her emotional life. Lest we should see this entirely in terms of the devastation wreaked upon women in heterosexual relationships, Kate Millett in *Sita*[17] depicts the same losing of the self in a lesbian relationship.

Scott's Susan feels she is nothing and hopes that by finding an outside shell she will become at least a parody of a person. The other heroines do have a veneer of autonomy in their lives but collapse inwardly when they engage in relationships which evoke their dependency and their longing to return to a fantasised blissful state of union with the other person.

What happens to women in intimate relationships is the province of Chapter 3 (see p.49). What I am concerned with is the way in which women often lack any sense of inner separation so that their identity crumbles when an intimate relationship touches them at a more primitive level. This illustrates the distinction made earlier between the conscious sense of identity and the unconscious level at which a woman may still be striving to merge with (or be a part of) her mother.

I want now to look at three women whom I have seen in therapy;* the experience of each highlights some of the difficulties women have in establishing a separate psychological identity. A combination of external circumstances, and conscious and unconscious processes brought these women to the point where their established modes of surviving were counter-productive and yet they could not find other ways of being in the world. They came to therapy when they found that the identities they had constructed to exclude or cope with certain conflicts were also preventing them from doing other things, causing them increasing frustration. In therapy we found that these identities were constructed around a lack of certain basic experiences, those of symbiosis with the mother and of development through a series of psychological phases necessary to the establishment of a separate identity. It would not be correct to describe these women's identities as false, but rather as defensive and restrictive.

---

* Details have been altered in the interest of confidentiality.

Angela

Angela's parents had fostered a child during World War II who stayed and became part of the family but Angela, conceived when her parents were reunited after the war, had a special position as her parents' first-born child of their own. Angela seemed to symbolise hope for the life her parents wanted to build together. From the start Angela was a disappointing baby. She was small and sickly and her mother found her hard to care for. She put on a brave front and tried to look satisfied but from early on what Angela saw in her mother's eyes was neediness. Unconsciously Angela took in the truth about her situation; she was there to satisfy her mother. While her parents struggled to build up a small painting and decorating business together, it was clear that her father could not satisfy her mother's emotional needs; that was Angela's job. The emotional situation was too precarious for Angela to learn about herself; to discover her own reflection through her mother and to learn gradually and safely that the world did not conform to her desires. She could not afford to try things out and know that someone would pick her up if her steps faltered; nor could she feel safe in expressing her disappointment if things did not turn out as she wanted them. Angela always had to test her mother's mood first. Very early on Angela developed an independent position. At her nursery she would refuse the offer of a special treat or stand outside the games. She often felt misunderstood by adults who took her apparently unassailable position at face value; she had put the longing part of herself aside and it seemed as if no one wanted to question that.

As Angela got older and more children were born, her parents' relationship deteriorated and her father left. This family split confirmed Angela's mental picture of her family. As she saw it, it wasn't that her mother was left holding the babies but that she, Angela, was left holding 'baby mother'. Her mother had a series of boyfriends who appeared to provide money but expected Angela's mother to carry on with them as though she had no responsibilities for children. Angela as the eldest girl kept the household going. She began to feel more and more desperate and could see no way out for herself but to leave home. She and a friend left Scotland secretly, hitched to London and managed to survive, squatting and gradually improving their living and working conditions. Angela appeared to be quite independent externally; leaving home was characteristic.

Angela came to therapy when she began to realise that as an adult, in her marriage and subsequent relationships, she was taking all the responsibility for keeping things going; accommodating other people's needs and in no way satisfying herself. She was repeating the role she had had in her family. She felt desperate, ministering to the needs of others, yet seemed quite unable to do anything to change her relationships. This suggested that she might be hanging on to her apparently independent responsible self for some hidden reason. While her mother had dealt with a similar emotional pattern by having Angela and unconsciously expressing her hidden needs in that relationship, Angela, in a different environment, was able to know that she needed therapy to help her understand her apparently self-defeating behaviour. She came to understand that she was protecting the very needy split-off infant part of herself, which in fantasy was still attached to her mother, and which had never had a chance to emerge, test reality and gradually develop into a separate sense of self. Her parents had been unable to create an environment where this was possible and Angela had responded to the situation by working very hard at keeping her needy infant part split off while developing her 'survival tactics'.

Mary

In Mary's family, as in Angela's, the common emotional division between mother and father, with mother carrying the feelings and father not engaging emotionally, left the mother feeling very needy and therefore unable to relate to her daughter as anything other than an extension of herself. In Mary's family, her mother carried the additional stress of having been almost forcibly moved from her own country to Britain. Angela had a semblance of mothering in that she was continuously cared for by her mother until her family split up when she was in her early teens. Mary's mother had what was diagnosed as a post-partum psychosis. Soon after Mary's birth, her mother was in and out of mental hospital and Mary was taken into care several times. Having many separations from her family, both physical and psychological, she developed a capacity to feel that what was happening to her was unreal. Her unconscious fantasy was that she could protect herself in this way.

The split in Mary's home encouraged this way of coping for it was an extreme version of a family where mother is 'a bit nervy' or over-emotional and father and the other males appear competent and unemotional. Mary's mother was defined as emotional and mad; her father and uncle were unemotional and clever. All the anxiety and disruption of being first-generation immigrants were 'carried' for the family by Mary's mother. Mary's brother identified with the men but Mary was 'mother's little girl'. In family turmoils Mary would always side with her mother. Her uncle played an important role in encouraging Mary and her brother to do well at school. Her uncle was also very much party to the family denial that there was anything upsetting about having a mother who suddenly collapsed or became unapproachable and disappeared for days or weeks.

Mary felt recognised as mother's little girl and as a clever schoolgirl but no one appeared to notice her adolescence. Sexuality was ignored. She got pregnant when she was sixteen and it was only through the intervention of her mother's social worker that her pregnancy was acknowledged and she had an abortion. She did not consciously feel anything about the experience but she began to find it harder and harder to leave the house.

She came to therapy when she had started college as a mature student and was finding it increasingly difficult to attend lectures and tutorials. The split she had built up between her intellectual and emotional life would not hold. The fantasy of being mother's little girl was not enough to sustain her emotionally. Something had to change. For Mary to look at the split between her intellectual and emotional sides and examine her relationship with her mother was inevitably going to be an arduous task in which she would have to recognise much that had been denied. She had internalised her family split so that while she apparently operated rationally and intellectually, she unconsciously felt at one with her very distressed mother. Yet she appeared to have an identity which was quite different from her mother's. Unconsciously she was terrified that her crazy part would emerge. In her fantasy she and her mother were still one person. This knowledge was both her life raft and her most carefully repressed and guarded secret. It was the only way she had found to protect her precarious connection with her mother who had neither been able to give her the initial safety and trust, nor been able to provide her with a safe background from which she could go through a process of separation. The price she paid was to maintain a hidden part which still held on to her mother's very particular view of the world. These two parts of herself, one very different from her mother, and the other (in Mary's fantasy) still inside her mother, were in conflict, and this manifested itself in her inability to do the thing she consciously most wanted to do; to study. Studying might come between her and mother; mother might be envious and might associate Mary with the men she had been damaged by. Mary might not be able to maintain the balance between the adult intellectual and the part of her which, in fantasy, was still a foetus in her mother's womb. Mary did not simply identify with her mother or fantasise a symbiotic relationship. Their early relationship had been so traumatic that her longing was to return to the womb. Mary had no experience which could allow her to begin the process of merging and then feeling strong enough to separate.

Evelyn

Evelyn's family were concerned with preserving their respectable image. They thought it normal not to show any strong feelings, especially negative ones like grief and anger. Her mother had had two stillborn babies before Evelyn was born but these losses were not acknowledged in the family. There was nothing in their social setting which suggested that mourning would be an appropriate response. When Evelyn was born her parents were very anxious about her.

Evelyn developed strange rashes and wheezes soon after she was born and it turned out that she had several allergies. Thus her early childhood was dominated by hospital visits and sickness. It seemed that much of the loving and caring she received related to being ill. She remembered her father searching the house for cool things to put on her face and arms to soothe her rashes. Being ill had its compensations: being the centre of attention, especially physical attention, without needing to feel a sense of guilt. At the same time it was constraining and frustrating. There were many things she was not allowed to do: go swimming, mix with other children, get over-tired, play with anything dirty – the list was endless.

Evelyn grew up with a very strong conscious sense that she needed attention; lots of it. She felt she didn't want to give attention to others. She didn't want to have children of her own to look after. She put a lot of effort into maintaining a series of complex extra-marital relationships. Yet she felt constantly frustrated. In her relationships she was attended to and looked after but after the initial excitement she was sexually bored. She also wanted to do exciting things in her life which she hardly dared contemplate for fear that they would upset her lovers and deprive her of the attention she got from being the 'little woman'.

The conflict between these two parts of herself became so intense and frustrating that she came to therapy desperate at the thought of continuing as she was but afraid of being well and powerful and of giving up her identity as a sick person. In her therapy she would have to find out why she was so locked into this sick identity and would have to struggle to establish a different sense of self. In spite of her overtly active sexual life she was internally stuck as mother's sick little girl, addicted to the physical care which had been her mother's substitute for a real capacity to relate to a healthy child. Her mother could not allow her to be a real/well person and she was too afraid of being alone to struggle against her mother's version of who she was.

Like Angela and Mary, Evelyn had never really experienced a relationship with her mother in which her needs as a healthy child were seen and understood; there had been no possibility of creating the illusion of omnipotence in which the infant can believe that she has only to whisper and mother comes running. Nor had Evelyn been able to develop from that early stage into a safe space where she could begin to explore her own capacities. For Evelyn there was no gradual path towards establishing a separate sense of self. Based on her early experience she could only see a gulf between a kind of addictive but unsatisfying attention and the terrifyingly dangerous excitement of an independent life.

These are three examples of women who, while apparently leading their own lives, are internally wedded to their mothers' visions of who they are. They do not know how to separate and establish their own identities at more than a superficial level. They are unable to discover their own desires as opposed to re-enacting some aspects of their parents' unconscious conflicts. They are not able to do this because they have not gone through the stages and experiences vital to moving from a symbiotic to a separate sense of self. This lack is in turn created within and reinforced by a society which does not have a cultural image of a separate woman.

A feminist re-reading of Winnicott

I use the work of D.W. Winnicott on the separation process as my starting point in the search for ways to connect the distorted reflection women see in the social mirror and the mirroring of the girl infant in her mother's eyes. This is because his work on the twilight zone between the internal fantasy world and the external environment suggests a way of conceptualising this meeting point without reducing the socio-political to the psychological or explaining away the processes of the internal world in sociological or political terms.[18]

It may seem surprising that, as a feminist, I should be so interested in his work since he is often seen as one of the psychoanalytic writers of the post-World War II era whose focus on the importance of the mother–child relationship was used to support the prevalent view that women should return home and look after their children.[19]

I have had a chequered and stormy relationship with his work. I have often found myself identifying so strongly either with the deprived infant or with the 'not-good-enough mother' that I have felt under attack. His often unstated ideological assumptions do affect his work as I will show. There is a tension between his keen awareness of the difficulties of being a mother and his inability fully to grasp the implications of this for women's lives.

I suggest that it is the very areas which Winnicott delineates in his account of the separation process which are crucial in forming female psychology. I have found Winnicott's account invaluable in understanding my therapy work but I have found it necessary to incorporate an understanding of the importance of gender which he ignores. I shall show how some of the phases Winnicott describes have a special meaning in the context of the mother–daughter relationship.

Winnicott sees the basis of successful separation as twofold. Firstly the infant needs a good experience of merging with her or his mother until s/he is ready to move out towards separation. Secondly it is equally important that the mother allows the infant to move outwards at its own gradual pace. The mother must be present for the growing infant but must also slowly reduce the amount that she intervenes so that the infant is able to do things alone, yet within a safe environment in which the mother can be turned to when necessary. She must be able to recognise the child's growing capacity to cope with the environment and hold back from intervening. The mother enables the child to begin to recognise its separate existence.

The first phase (the merged or symbiotic phase) starts towards the end of pregnancy and continues into the first weeks of the infant's life. Winnicott terms this the period of 'primary maternal preoccupation'. 'By and large mothers do in one way or another identify themselves with the baby that is growing within them, and in this way they achieve a very powerful sense of what the baby needs. This is a projective identification. This identification with the baby lasts for a certain length of time after parturition and then gradually loses significance.'[20] Winnicott recognises the peculiar nature of this state of primary maternal preoccupation, which he describes as a 'normal illness' from which the mother will recover. He suggests that to achieve this state the mother begins to turn her attention in on herself quite early in pregnancy. In so doing she 'shifts some of her sense of self on to the baby that is growing within her'.[21] He also recognises that 'an adoptive mother or any woman who can be ill in the sense of primary maternal preoccupation may be in a position to adapt well enough on account of having some capacity for identification with the baby'.[22]

What is described is familiar to us both in everyday life and in therapy. Those who have had babies or been close to a mother–baby couple will have noticed the way in which a very special atmosphere seems to pervade those early weeks. The mother does often seem to be in a strange state and very vulnerable. This stage is not necessarily idyllic. As some of the mothers whom Ann Oakley interviewed for her book *From Here to Maternity*[23] described it: 'I lived in a permanent haze ... I can't really remember what I did the first day. All I can remember is crying. I was and he was.' (p.141) 'Everything is absolutely completely different. I mean I look at the news and there could be a third world war and it's not really important at the moment.' (p.163) 'I used to be self-centred and I'm not any more; I haven'ɩ got the time to be. I'm thinking of her all the time. What time she'll be waking up, what I must do. I don't think about myself any more.' (p.163)

In what sense is it true to say that the mother feels what the baby is feeling? Winnicott says that the mother's capacity to feel with her baby is related to her own experience of being mothered. If her own mothering was dominated by unmet needs then she is likely either to withdraw from too close contact with her baby's feelings for fear of her own distress being reactivated (as Evelyn's mother did, substituting nursing care for an empathetic relationship); or she may regress beyond the ill-defined point of normality and be unable to distinguish clearly between herself and her baby (Mary's mother regressed to the point where she became psychotic). When the mother and baby are merged the mother feels what her baby is feeling but at the same time is aware that there is a distinction between her and the baby. The baby cannot distinguish between herself and her mother at first and experiences the mother's breast as an extension of herself. She is not able to communicate her needs explicitly to the mother. Mother has to feel when her baby is uncomfortable, hungry, cold or sleepy.

Winnicott's account of primary maternal preoccupation is illuminating but also limited. Some feminist writers have argued that mothering a girl infant and being 'at one' with her is different and unconsciously more threatening and powerful than merging with a boy infant.* Further, Winnicott grossly underestimates the long-term implications of the capacity to experience 'primary maternal preoccupation' for women's psychology. His description of that capacity as 'normal illness'[24] is appealing but he does not really spell the metaphor out. An implicit reference is being made to a disease model of illness, where an infection simply comes and goes from a person's body. There is no process of preparation or build-up to the illness and once cured the person is seen as being essentially the same as before. Primary maternal preoccupation is not really analogous to this (quite apart from the question of whether this model of illness is valid anyway). Winnicott recognises the importance of the mother's own early infantile experience in her subsequent capacity to mother, which implies that primary maternal preoccupation does not hit the mother like a measles germ. Yet he draws no conclusions from this. Nor does he see the continuity between the capacity for maternal preoccupation and the way in which identification with others is a central feature of women's personality. In contrast to this, Chodorow, writing from a feminist perspective, sees the capacity for primary maternal preoccupation as a constant and central feature of women's personalities.[25]

---

* This will be looked at in detail in the next section.

If the 'ideal' form of primary maternal preoccupation existed, a psychologically separate mother would be able to identify with her baby and yet maintain her own boundaries. However the difficulties that women have in achieving psychological separation suggest to me that the experience of primary maternal preoccupation is more likely to be continuous with women's ongoing lack of psychological separation. Winnicott fails to see that women's psychological structure is reinforced by their economic and social experience – the *relative* absence of adult separate social identities for women. It is his lack of any political perspective on gender which limits his understanding of women's psychology.

The context of the early relationship

Yet Winnicott provides a basis for the feminist development of object relations theory. He sees himself as having a more developed awareness of the importance of the infant's environment than did his psychoanalytic predecessors. He writes, 'both Freud and Klein avoided the full implication of dependence and therefore of the environmental factor'.[26] What he means by environment is in the first place the 'skin' in which the mother contains her baby; he recognised that another support system was necessary to maintain the mother–baby couple. This second skin is usually provided by the father or others close to the mother and allows the mother to regress to the degree necessary for her to be in touch with the baby's needs. Thus a mother's capacity to merge with her infant is also dependent on the environment.

He is aware of the culturally relative nature of our child-rearing arrangements. He understands that the individual will have within herself elements normally attributed to the opposite sex and that these need recognition. He also knows that women are oppressed and sometimes treated with cruelty but as a man with no political analysis of gender he cannot take this knowledge into the centre of his work. The closest he comes is in his suggestion that we might alter men's attitudes to women through studying mothering and beginning to combat men's unconscious fears of women in this way.[27]

Mirroring

A crucial part of the earliest phase is the mirroring of the baby in the mother's face. If all is well the baby gazes into the mother's face and sees itself reflected. If the mother is too preoccupied the 'mirror' reflects the mother back to the baby. The baby will then have to learn to predict its mother's mood instead of focusing on itself and its own image. 'The mother's face is not then a mirror. So perception takes the place of apperception, perception takes the place of that which might have been the beginning of a significant exchange with the world, a two-way process in which self-enrichment alternates with the discovery of meaning in the world of seen things.'[28]

Just as in the introduction we looked at the difficulty for an adult woman of seeing her face reflected in the mirror, so there are particular difficulties for the mother in mirroring her daughter. Winnicott illustrates his article on mirroring with an example of a woman who, 'had to be her own mother. If she had had a daughter she would surely have found great relief, but perhaps a daughter would have suffered because of having too much importance in correcting her mother's uncertainty about her own mother's sight of her.'[29]

I think that this is the task which daughters in our society are required to do for mothers who are emotionally deprived and lacking in the social mirroring of their reality. The daughters themselves, therefore, are not likely to receive adequate reflections back from their mothers.

Omnipotent fantasies and the graduated failure of adaptation

Having recognised the significance of the earliest phase Winnicott is at pains to emphasise the importance of the mother's capacity to respond to the infant's maturation by a graduated failure of adaptation. 'There is a very subtle distinction between the mother's understanding of her infant's need based on empathy, and her change over to an understanding based on something in the infant or small child that indicates need.'[30] Thus while an empathic caretaker is necessary for a healthy start to a baby's life, if this empathy is continued beyond where it is necessary it can prevent the baby from developing a confidence in its own demands and a capacity to relate to others. This is different from the popular image of the 'good mother' intuiting her child's needs before the child has even articulated them. Mother's task is now to be available when needed but to draw back and allow the infant autonomy so that s/he may maintain an illusion of omnipotence; that it controls the world around and that it creates the objects to which it relates. Thus at first the infant does not experience itself except as part of the mother; then an illusion is created by the mother that if the infant has a desire it will be met. This cushions the infant's first awareness of the outside world. It is then the mother's task to allow the infant to come to an awareness of the independent existence of the outside at an appropriate rate.

This is a difficult task for the mother. Perhaps more difficult than Winnicott recognised because he did not see how the psychology of the mother was permanently less 'bounded' than that of most men. Thus the mother has the job of introducing her baby to something she herself does not fully grasp. She may be highly ambivalent about letting go of her infant for merging may still be the only form of closeness she can conceive of. She may have more difficulty in disentangling herself from a daughter. Being the same as her daughter it is hard to allow her to explore; either the mother does not let her daughter take any risks or, in order to let go of her daughter, she finds herself having to withdraw, to put up false boundaries. Marilyn Lawrence in her account of anorexia[31] describes how mother and daughter cannot let go of each other. The daughter eventually stakes out a claim for herself by taking total control of her food intake. Marilyn Lawrence relates this

specifically to the failure to work through the phase of omnipotent fantasy. Margaret Mahler's empirical work[32] seems to
confirm this viewpoint: she suggests that it is at the point of
giving up fantasies of omnipotence that girls experience a lot
of difficulty and are likely to regress. Of course this is socially
reinforced in our expectation that girls will not be as successful
as boys in their manipulation of the world around them.

Transitional objects and phenomena; the concept of play

So infants need to move from being merged with mother,
through a period when they fantasise they have total control
over the outside world (which in their fantasy they have created)
to a gradual realisation that people do exist separately from
them and that therefore they too have a separate existence. To
mediate this transition the child may select an object to which
she attaches special significance.[33] The classic example is the
child's special blanket or rag – the 'baa' – which the mother
allows to remain under the child's control. This object does
exist in the real world; for instance it can get lost or hidden by
another child so that it is not under magical control like a fantasised object, yet it is not totally outside control as a person
is. The mother colludes with the child's view of the object as
special; she will help to find it, make sure it is always there at
crucial times and agree not to wash it so that it retains its special
smells. This object can give a child a safe mid-ground in which
to practise relating to the world outside without having to risk
completely giving up fantasised control. If it does not success-
fully negotiate this transition the child will repress its fears of
losing control and will unconsciously remain in the phase of
omnipotence, while appearing to be operating as an individual
in the adult world. Winnicott suggests that moving into the
transitional area (the mid-ground mentioned above), the arena
of play and creativity, is what makes people feel that life is
worth living. In his clinical examples he describes patients who
apparently have fulfilled lives and yet experience themselves as
quite unfulfilled and depressed. They have been living without

engaging this live creative part. He does not see any difference between men's and women's experience. He says specifically, 'there is no noticeable difference between boy and girl in their use of the original "not-me" possession,'[34] but that gradually boys move on to playing with 'hard objects' and girls 'recreate families'. Girls and boys may choose the same first transitional object but it is unlikely that they will use them in the same way. Girls find it harder than boys to move on to the creative arena and it may be that they use their transitional objects as comforters, as ways of fantasising that they are back with their mothers, rather than as potential objects which they can control by direct manipulation.

It is the process of trial and error involved in playing, in the constant reworking and practising of manipulations, events and situations which allows the child to move from the arena of magic and wishing, to the arena of real cause and effect. Through play the child can come to recognise in a safe way that objects may exist outside the area of its omnipotent control.

> In the state of confidence that grows up . . . the baby begins to enjoy experiences based on a 'marriage' of the omnipotence of intrapsychic processes with the baby's control of the actual . . . I call this a playground because play starts here. The playground is a potential space between the mother and the baby or joining mother and baby – the thing about playing is always the precariousness of the interplay of personal psychic reality and the experience of control of actual objects. This is the precariousness of magic itself, magic that arises in intimacy in a relationship that is found to be reliable.[35]

A girl busy picking up signals from others, reading her mother's mood from a glance, not having been let go of by her mother at a gradual pace, does not really feel safe enough to enter this playground that Winnicott describes. Thus she has not really been able to move through the preparatory phases to the point where she can see herself existing separately from other objects. Winnicott suggests that the test for the child is to risk venting its destructive feelings on an object and discovering that the object can survive, thus proving its independent existence. This is also likely to pose difficulties for girls whose angry and destructive feelings are often repressed, especially in relation to mother. The daughter is likely to fantasise that her mother will never survive her rage and therefore will never test it out.

The girl may unconsciously maintain a fantasy of her omnipotent control over reality while in her daily life she is busy making herself safe and fitting in with others rather than being able to involve herself in the activities of play and thence in real control and activity in the world.

It is this very area of play in which the social and psychological converge that requires special attention for women in therapy so that women do get a safe space to play in and can begin to acknowledge themselves.

Feminist theorists

It is curious that Winnicott did not appear to differentiate between boys and girls in their maturational processes when he was so supremely aware of the importance of the maternal environment. Yet Freud, Klein and other psychoanalytic writers on the 'femininity' issue in the thirties had all addressed themselves to the idea that for girls the pre-oedipal period was both longer and possibly more significant than for boys. Freud wrote, 'We get the impression that we cannot understand women unless we appreciate this phase of their pre-oedipal attachment to their mother.'[36]

The debate about women's psychology in the thirties was partly carried on by women psychoanalysts who were concerned about the social position of women. Similarly the feminist concern now is to understand what effect living in patriarchy has upon a girl's psychological development. For some these questions are asked not only out of theoretical interest but also out of a desire for changes in practice. Others believe that 'Psychoanalysis should not subscribe to ideas about how men and women do or should live as sexually differentiated bengs but instead it should analyse how they come to be such beings in the first place.'[37] Later we shall see how the type of explanation which a theorist offers is intimately connected with her views on the nature of theory and its relationship to politics and science. These are topics which we must acknowledge as being relevant to our understanding of the differences between feminist theorists while we shall not be able to explore them fully here.

There are two significant contemporary strands of feminist psychoanalytic writing which bear on the topic of psychological separation: the object relations theorists, who follow on from Winnicott[38] in concentrating on the early relationship between infant and mother, but focus on the mother–daughter relationship as a crucial locus of internalised oppression; and those feminists who have taken up the Lacanian re-reading of Freud and are interested in how sexual difference is constructed. Both draw on notions of feminism as well as on their psychoanalytic predecessors – object relations theory concentrating much attention on the earliest phase of life, and Lacan seeing the centrality of gender identity. I shall take the work of Chodorow and Eichenbaum and Orbach to represent the former group and the work of Mitchell as one of the best known, though not necessarily totally representative, of the latter.

The feminist development of object relations theory suggests that at an unconscious level the dyadic unit of mother–daughter is not broken into, while Mitchell defines differentiation in terms of the father who, 'stands in the position of the third term that *must* break the asocial dyadic unit of mother and child'.[39]

Using Winnicott's model of the unconscious processes which must take place for psychological separation to be achieved, I have shown how social and psychological factors interact to make this a problematic process for mothers and daughters. The issue is then not so much the absence of father representing society but rather the presence of father's society, that is, patriarchy and its effect on the psychological development of girls.

Feminist object relations theory

I want to restate two assumptions that underlie this approach. One is that the nature of the relationship between mother and infant will be affected by the fact that the mother is a woman in a patriarchal society and is contending with the oppression that this implies. Secondly, that the sex of the infant and the mother's unconscious feelings about girls and boys (in turn affected by patriarchy) will have a bearing on how the mother and baby relate.

Chodorow, as a sociologist, uses object relations theory to explain why it is that women keep on doing the 'mothering'. While Winnicott saw primary maternal preoccupation as a temporary phase, Chodorow suggests that it is central to the psychic structuring of girls in our society. Mother and daughter share an unresolved inner object world in which they maintain an unconscious fantasy of continuity with one another. Neither of them is able to move towards separation. Women are thus prepared to 'experience the empathy and lack of reality sense needed by a cared for infant'.[40] In other words, mothering reproduces itself. While Mitchell sees the father as the *necessary* third point in the triangle, to enable differentiation, for Chodorow the *actual* third point in the triangle is the daughter's new baby, when the daughter herself becomes a mother.

Chodorow uses existing case material to infer the crucial significance of the early mother–daughter symbiotic relationship. She suggests that 'the girl becomes the self of the mother's fantasy'[41] but does not have the material to draw on to show how this happens. Instead she argues that the different ways in which boys and girls resolve their oedipal conflicts account for the girls' 'more conflictual and less resolved inner world'.[42] Eichenbaum and Orbach, using their own clinical experience, develop an account of the earliest phase of the mother–daughter relationship which suggests that this is the crucial formative phase for girls and that the oedipal difference is more superficial.[43] (The implication for therapy with women is that it will focus on the symbiotic phase.) They spell out more precisely what is involved for the daughter in becoming the self of the mother's fantasy. The mother looking at her infant daughter is, as Winnicott says, drawn into identification with her; seeing her helpless daughter she unconsciously projects into her all her own feelings of despair, hopelessness, rage about her own disappointments and lack of nurturing. The infant girl expressing her needs comes to represent the repressed part of the mother. The mother, reminded of feelings she cannot tolerate in herself, unconsciously pushes the girl away. At other times she deals with the conflict aroused in her by giving the infant what she herself unconsciously desires, even if it is not appropriate for the baby. Perhaps there is also another element involved; unconscious guilt at rejecting her daughter and an attempt to make reparations. Thus a push–pull dynamic is set up in this earliest stage of the mother–daughter relationship. The mother wants specially to love and nurture her daughter because she identifies with her and recognises her daughter's need. She sublimates her own neediness into nurturing her daughter; then when the restimulation becomes too painful she pushes her away. Thus the daughter does not have a very secure experience of symbiosis; her needy part is split off and repressed so that it is easier for the mother to cope with; the daughter is beginning to be formed in her mother's image.

In therapeutic work we see the process Eichenbaum and Orbach describe in the transference relationship between woman therapist and client. I first noticed this pattern in my own therapy. After a session in which I felt very dependent and tearful and had made new connections for myself, I was then acutely aware in the next session of my therapist's presence. I took gestures she made as critical, felt very uncomfortable in 'my' seat and got into that peculiar state of self-consciousness where blowing my nose seemed like a major decision. The whole session seemed to be a step backwards after the previous positive hour. It was as if in the transference I saw my therapist as the push–pull mother. Looking back I feel sure that she did not change from one time to another. I assumed the response and reacted appropriately, becoming very anxious about how I might have disturbed her. In my own work I have found similar patterns; a client who was just beginning to feel dependent suddenly found all sorts of excuses not to come to therapy. When I suggested that unconsciously she was frightened of feeling dependent on me she laughed it off. Gradually it became clear that she thought I was not really interested in seeing her. As so often happens she had particularly interpreted the holiday break in this way. We were then able to relate this to the assumption that she was making unconsciously that I would withdraw as soon as I felt her dependency.

Similar conclusions (based on her experience as a therapist) about the difficulties mothers have in mothering daughters in the symbiotic phase and the consequences for the adult woman's psychology are reached by Flax.[44] She also thinks that women long to return to the fantasised symbiotic union with mother which they feel they never really had. She summarises the difficulties as follows. In the early mother–daughter relationship there are no boundaries. Mother's own ambivalence about being a woman affects her feelings towards her daughter. Mother has more internal conflict in relation to her daughter because her identification with the baby girl restimulates her own early experience and may come out in her desire to be mothered by her daughter. This is remarkably similar to some of Eichenbaum's and Orbach's observations. They too write of the mother being the daughter's first child. Chodorow sees the daughter as acquiring her capacity to mother through the unboundedness of her relationship to her own mother and her mother's need to be mothered.

Flax also mentions the possibility that the mother may be anxious lest her physical closeness to her daughter will awaken repressed incestuous wishes. This is interesting in the light of the criticism by Ryan[45] that sexuality and particularly the sexual feelings between mother and daughter are ignored by Chodorow and Eichenbaum and Orbach.

We have therefore one feminist perspective which suggests that women's separation difficulties go back to their experience of the symbiotic phase and that this can be understood most clearly in terms of the social and emotional deprivation of the mothers (women) rearing these children and the problems arising out of being the same sex. All three return to Freud in their emphasis on the importance of the symbiotic phase but they see this as being only one part of what keeps the daughter tied to the mother's apron strings.

Analysis of a woman by a woman: feminist and non-feminist compared

A similar perspective is reached in an article by Pines on women who have suffered from infantile eczema. Her observations seem entirely consistent with the feminist perspective. She reminds us that a basic disturbance in the mother–infant relationship is 'renewed with every transitional phase of the life cycle'.[46] The history of these particular girl infants means that they have had physical soothing of their eczema substituted for emotional soothing. Pines points to the vitally important experiences they have missed out on. She implies that the infant's skin irritation stems from the mother's inability to contain the infant's negativity at an emotional level. Not having a mother who can contain her anxiety the infant cannot introject that containment and therefore does not develop the sense of self and object contained in separate skins. Eichenbaum and Orbach argue that mothers in general cannot contain little girls' anxieties.

Although the mother–daughter relationship is expressed through special physical treatment for eczema, the mother will often be disappointed in the baby's body so that the girl with eczema will not get the kind of narcissistic reinforcement she needs to begin to separate from her mother. It may be that all girls are deprived to some extent of 'an adequate maternal mirroring response of admiration for the child's body'.[47] We could understand this in terms of a mother's ambivalence to her daughter as being the same as herself or, as Mitchell might see it, as the mother's counter-identification with the daughter's lack (of a penis).

Writing about the special nature of the relationship between the woman analyst and her woman patient, Pines suggests that the woman analyst's biological capacity to be a mother evokes primitive transference feelings in her patients arising from what she terms 'partial maternal deprivation'. She also notes both the longing for intimate contact and the fear of being swallowed up (see Eichenbaum's and Orbach's chapter on Separation and intimacy, p.49). She suggests that in spite of a woman having the outward manifestations of an adult heterosexual life she *may* lack internal individuation. Eichenbaum and Orbach agree with Pines in seeing that the girl has not experienced herself as being emotionally contained and has therefore split off and repressed that part of herself which is still tied to her mother. They suggest that the part of the girl which appears to be maturing and relating to the outside world is split off from this much more primitive aspect. Thus there is not so much a process of unconscious internal change as a kind of donning of sophisticated clothing which does not fundamentally alter the 'baby' underwear. It is not that one part is more real than the other but rather that they co-exist in an often uncomfortable and destructive way.

They suggest that this split-off part constantly influences the girl or woman in her everyday life and sense of herself. Thus she may identify with her internalised message from her mother about the dangerous nature of the world outside and this unconscious knowledge may then be used to influence the placatory way in which she relates to others. She must live as they want her to and all her energy goes into being sensitive to them, not into acknowledging what she might want; her sexuality is for pleasing others rather than for her own satisfaction. The external world reinforces these images at increasingly subtle levels. While at one time popular images of women showed them in only a limited number of situations and in conventionally serving or sexy roles, we now have images of apparently 'free' and 'independent' women. Yet if we examine these more closely, as Roz Coward does in *Female Desire*,[48] we see how they are but new glosses on old pressures to conformity. Thus the internal world of the girl, formed within society, is maintained in its female form by continuing influence from outside. What I am positing is not a simplistic learning theory account of girls' conditioning but rather a complex web of interrelating threads running between inner and outer worlds. Social situation and early experience formed within society.

affect the child's fantasy life in ways that emerge slowly in the therapy relationship.

Mitchell: separation and the construction of sexual difference

A point of connection between Juliet Mitchell and the other feminist theorists we have been looking at is in their criticism of object relations theory for not taking gender sufficiently into account in the earliest formation of the human being. Mitchell writes, '[They] concentrated attention on the mother and the sexually undifferentiated child, leaving the problem of sexual distinction as a subsidiary that is somehow not bound up with the very formation of the subject.'[49] While I and the writers we have just looked at try to rectify this by re-examining the mother—daughter relationship within the context of patri-archy, Mitchell argues that a fundamental error has been made: 'this is the price paid for the reorientation to the mother and the neglect of the father whose prohibition in Freud's theory can alone represent the mark that distinguishes boys and girls.'[50]

Behind this lie some assumptions about the nature of the unconscious and its relationship to becoming a human (by which I think she means entering society). At the outset there is no male or female persona; the question for psychoanalysis is how the non-differentiated subject becomes the human man or woman, for to become human is to take up a position as either man or woman. Being human is defined as being within the structure of the law represented by the father. The rela-tionship between mother and child thus has to be seen within the framework of 'the structure established by the position of the father'.[51] Becoming human means recognising a lack and for the girl this means lack of the phallus; she recognises that she is like mother in having no phallus and different from father. Thus she recognises herself as a woman within the framework of the castration complex.

For Mitchell the recognition of not having a phallus is essential to the female psyche; that is what being a woman in patriarchy is about. She is aware of the power relations involved; this is what she is theorising. What Mitchell says is illuminating in that it makes us see that, whatever our development, it takes place within a culture in which phallus equals having and no phallus defines a person as not having. Yet the implication of this level of theory is unchangeability. The question of whether we could have a society in which having/not having was defined in non-phallic terms is not seen as relevant. Nor (as Janet Sayers points out)[52] is the question of *un*successful taking up of the women's role at issue.

Yet Mitchell thinks that object relations theory takes men and women as given and is asking questions about human development at quite a different level; taking a biologically given sexual identity such theorists then look at how the baby interacts with real objects and its fantasies of those objects in its development towards maturity. This she connects to a question about whether the human environment has been 'good enough' for the baby to develop; implicitly she is suggesting that there is a humanistic avoidance of the true and terrifying nature of the unconscious. While this may be true of some psychoanalysis within the object relations tradition it does not seem to me to be necessarily the case. Moreover I am made suspicious by the insinuation that what she/Lacan/Freud are doing is deeper, and is bypassing mere empiricism. Mitchell comes to Lacan/ Freud from an Althusserian background, taking a stance on the science of Marxism which is not unlike the stance on the science of psychoanalysis. The positions are similarly seductive. We can stand back and examine the true structure of society, class struggle or the unconscious. The offer of 'a science which takes up a position which is superior to experience thereby situating us outside the struggles in society observing the process'[53] is appealing to intellectuals (and even to psychotherapists). Yet this contradicts the very essence of psychoanalytic knowledge which is to be precisely inside (learning from transference and counter-transference) and outside (interpreting and theorising) at the same time. Nor does it allow for the ways in which our own theoretical work is a part of the struggle for change waged at conscious and unconscious levels.

Conclusions

We appear to have two opposed positions: the feminist object relations line in which the girl/woman's separation issues involve the negotiation of the mother–daughter relationship, and Mitchell's argument that this avoids the issue and that what is central is the posing of a 'third term' which breaks into the asocial dyadic relationship. If we recognise, as Mitchell does, that the third term is not literally the father, but what the father symbolises as a recognition of the subject's existence in a world in which she is not merged with mother (i.e. an accepting of the loss or absence of the breast) then it seems to me that we are entering common ground. For the dyadic relationship in the work of Eichenbaum and Orbach is not asocial. Their account is precisely an attempt to show how society breaks into it from the start. Following this, my work on separation shows what is involved for a girl infant in accepting and integrating the loss of the breast and its concomitant – the possibility of acting in the world.

The presence of the father as 'patriarchy' is central to the work of Eichenbaum and Orbach. It is within the patriarchal context that the mother acquires her particular identity and therefore has the kind of relationship we have described with her daughter. They point out the way in which the father's relative physical and emotional absence both contextualises and yet reinforces the mother–daughter relationship. Lastly and crucially Eichenbaum and Orbach point out that it may be easier for boys to separate from mother, not only because they have father to identify with but also because they can hope to grow up and have another woman to nurture them. For girls, adaptation to a heterosexual society appears to mean replacing being nurtured by becoming a nurturer. This is the meaning of Chodorow's triangle – mother, daughter, baby.

Politically we may challenge the social and economic manifestations of this triangle, ranging from the lack of nursery provision to the low pay in some of the predominantly women's caring professions such as nursing, physiotherapy and primary school teaching. In therapy we work on the woman's internal world to create an environment in which she can explore both the early symbiotic relationship and then move on through the other phases in the development of a differentiated self. In doing this we will have to maintain a constant awareness of the way in which the external world may reinforce the woman's own fears of change.

Bringing a feminist perspective on separation into the therapy relationship with women

I now want to look at some of the issues which I have found important in my work as a therapist with women, drawing on the ideas of Winnicott and different feminist theorists. I try in my work to see the interweaving of social and economic, conscious and unconscious in a way which recognises the contradictory nature of women's experience and how this affects their journey towards 'separateness'. Therapy is not a straightforward process but is marked by much to-ing an fro-ing, wanting and not wanting to change. It is also a more painful process than I am going to be able to convey.

I will look in some detail at the three women I have already described and will generalise to the unconscious experience of many other women: though there are crucial differences of class and race between women, it is the case that many women have far too little experience of emotional dependency. While focusing on neediness I would not however want to fall into the trap of repeating one of the experiences that makes separation so difficult for girls: the fact that there are so few explicit or validating images of separateness for women. I hope also to dispel the misconception that a feminist view of therapy offers a kind of perfect symbiosis within the reparative therapy relationship.

As we will see, each of the three women needed to reproduce the process of separation within the therapy relationship. At every phase the woman had to work through again the particular difficulties which prevented her from resolving earlier contradictions and moving on to a different psychological level. Before she can begin to separate she needs to experience her dependency; she looks to the therapist for mirroring, fantasises herself as omnipotent and needs to be given a safe space within which to test out her developing autonomy. She needs to move between fantasy and reality and discover that she can exist and allow others to exist. She also tests out her therapist's capacity to survive her attacks and discover that her destructive fantasies do not actually destroy the other person. The relationship between woman client and therapist often reflects the mother–child relationship. The client repeatedly feels that the therapist is like her mother and the therapist in turn often finds herself having feelings which may only be explicable in terms of unconscious communication from the client to the therapist. Thus, focusing on transference and counter-transference is crucial to the work.

Angela, Mary and Evelyn

The social dimension
I stated earlier that the social is inextricably interwoven with the psychological in the developing psyche of the child. However, some aspects of the social situations of these women and their families were especially significant, both in preventing separation and in bringing them to therapy. Two of the women came from working-class families and one from a lower-middle-class background. One woman was the daughter of first generation immigrants, another had left her home in Scotland. All three had used the availability of some kind of further education to make significant changes in their life situations. All three had used welfare state benefits and developments in the abortion/contraception services to alter what might otherwise have been a life dominated by child-bearing.

All three had been influenced by feminism; while not necessarily defining themselves as feminists they had been affected by other women who were challenging the experiences and possibilities open to women.

For each of these women the material changes they were able to make in their lives were important. On the one hand they opened up the time and resources within which change can seem like a possibility, where exploring the unconscious seemed like a risk they could afford to take. On the other hand, the possibilities which these changes opened up also intensified each woman's awareness of her lack of inner autonomy: expectations were raised but the reality was disappointing. The experience is similar to that described by Lynne Segal in her paper in *Sex and Love*. Feminists had an initial period of optimism over the possibility of changing their sexual experience, but this then gave way to years of silence on the subject. Only recently has a start been made in exploring the 'things we would rather avoid, masochism, self-objectification, domination, guilt, hostility and envy'.[54] It is the combination of potential and disappointment which often brings women to therapy.

Contrast the social situation and norms of Angela, Mary and Evelyn with those within which their mothers lived and brought them up. If Angela's mother had had more of a sense of the possibility of her own desires being *recognised*, would she have imbued Angela with such devastating psychic importance? If Mary's mother had not lived in a family with such an extreme form of sexual division between the emotional and non-emotional, which was supported by local social norms, would she have gone 'crazy'? If Evelyn's mother had lived in a society where grieving had a real place would she have been more able to mourn the loss of her two stillborn babies and then been more able to have a direct relationship with Evelyn? The limitations of these women's lives directly affected their daughters' earliest experience and we shall see how they were incorporated into the daughters' problems with separation.

The earliest phase: primary maternal preoccupation and symbiosis

Again and again in their therapy all three women returned to their longing to be understood by me without having to explain or tell me anything. They wanted me to be like a mother in tune with her baby's needs because they are as one. Yet what they often felt was that the only way to be at one with me was to accommodate to what they thought I wanted. Mary had always identified with her mother and this she transferred to me; wanting to be like me in all kinds of ways, from dressing alike to dying her hair black and to wanting to move into my house. If she could be me then she would not have to cope with the comings and goings which reminded her so painfully of the extreme uncertainty of her early childhood. For Mary it was as if mirroring was reversed; looking to her mother to mirror her, all she saw was her mother. A mother will unconsciously demand support from her daughter but this involves recognising her daughter's presence. Mary's mother was so often out of touch with reality that she did not realise Mary was there. Much of the work in her therapy was acknowledging her distress at not being seen.

The lack of mirroring came out clearly in Angela and Evelyn's therapy. Angela felt that she constantly had to measure what she was saying about herself against her perception of my distress-level – what she thought I could cope with. No matter how many sessions we had in which she would weep, apparently talking about her deep unhappiness, she did not really feel that I had taken in what she was saying. She complained that it was useless going on talking about how miserable she felt. It didn't change anything. It was only when we recognised that a part of her was always considering me and that she was going through the motions of therapy to test out what she could say to me, that we understood that she was not feeling heard or seen in the real sense of being 'mirrored'. Linking this to her early experience of gazing into her mother's eyes and seeing her mother's distress helped her to understand that she was seeing me as a woman and therefore as inevitably like her mother.

For Evelyn the issue was different. She did not feel she had to take care of me but rather assumed that I would not see her inner world at all; I would relate only to the external Evelyn. The assumption was that I would do a good professional job. She thought she had to work hard to make me notice her, whether through wearing clothes that she thought would make her stand out at the WTC, doing outrageous things or just talking loudly. She had literally to make sure she was seen and heard. She also found it very difficult to accept that I was not going to respond to her by looking after her practically. She was contemptuous about my lack of a medical training so that I could not comment on her illness from anything other than a psychological perspective. Nor would I come and cook her dinner for her. She managed to find a way in which she could, indirectly, get some 'practical' feeding from me. The WTC has a kitchenette where people can make hot drinks and where there is a tin of biscuits. She would always come into a session ostentatiously holding her coffee and dip her biscuits in, relishing every mouthful. It seemed that she could get more nourishment from the food and drink than she could from the emotional content of our sessions. We began to connect this way of seeing our relationship with the way in which Evelyn's mother had appeared to be very attentive to her physical needs as a sick child yet had also avoided contact with her as a baby. Her husband and her mother were both quite cold, withholding people. Evelyn's mother never really allowed herself to move into that state of primary maternal preoccupation; she defended herself against her daughter. So there was no symbiosis, no mirroring, but rather a job to be done. In the early days of her therapy Evelyn found holiday breaks almost intolerable because the only safety she could glean from the therapy relationship came from being in the same room as me. She had virtually no sense of what it meant to have a relationship involving communication. As we recognised this our relationship changed so that my seeing and hearing what she felt was something she could take in and use as a crucial part of her therapy.

The inadequate or non-existent mirroring which these daughters received from their mothers was connected with the mothers' situations and experiences. The lack of emotional sustenance in their own lives and the social and economic situations in which they lived meant that they were thrown into relationships with daughters who simply restimulated precisely those parts of their own lives and emotions which were unconsciously most distressing to them. It is not surprising that they either demanded that their daughters meet their emotional needs, failed to perceive the reality of their daughters' existence or fobbed them off with a kind of ersatz attention.

Omnipotence

Winnicott suggests that as it moves from the earliest symbiotic relationship the infant learns to demand attention. At first the infant fantasises that s/he is omnipotent because each demand appears to be met. Then gradually s/he comes to realise that the world is not as controllable as it seemed at first. By the time this truth has gradually dawned, it is not intolerable because the child has sufficient capacity to act upon the world to prevent the relationship with her mother from being unbearably threatening.

I think that there may be some difference between the omnipotent fantasies of boys and girls that is connected with the particular difficulties that mother and daughter experience in the symbiotic phase. This is reinforced by the way in which overt power is not seen as 'feminine' in our society. Angela's way of getting some illusion of power for herself was one of the most common. She gained some sense of control through withdrawing her own needs (in response to her mother's neediness and demand to be looked after). She avoided feeling vulnerable before people who might let her down, through taking care of others. In her fantasy she dealt with the impact my life had on her (for example, changing her times, taking my holidays at times which were inconvenient for her) by withdrawing, missing sessions and devaluing our relationship. By attempting not to let me upset her, she was able to maintain the illusion that she was in control. We were able to see that this was how she had dealt with things that did not conform to her desires as far back as she could remember. Mary too had a fantasy of her omnipotence, which was double-edged. Unconsciously she believed that she had driven her mother crazy; thus she was not the tiny frail victim of her mother's breakdown and her father's incapacity to sustain a close relationship. She was the powerful cause of all their troubles. While this protected her from the awful feelings of being deserted and her acute separation anxiety, it left her feeling that she was a deeply destructive person. In her therapy she found it extremely difficult to begin to test this fantasy out. She was afraid to explore her 'destructive' and attacking feelings towards me but was equally scared of experiencing her vulnerability and pain. Little by little our relationship gave her the space to explore the possibility of letting go of her fantasy image of herself as omnipotent and destructive, and to experience her pain in manageable doses. She came to see that she could survive her pain.

Evelyn's omnipotence was also two-sided; illness allowed her to control others but also barred her from participating in the life of healthy people. She felt stifled by receiving the care she demanded. Thus what appeared to be a capacity to get attention at will was in fact only the capacity to get attention she didn't want.

None of these women had omnipotent fantasies as Winnicott describes them in which all their needs were met. The form that their omnipotent fantasies took coloured the rest of the separation process.

Transition
The therapy session with its somewhat formal structure and clear boundaries can provide a space which allows a woman to shift aspects of herself while maintaining her fantasy of having control until she can afford to give the fantasy up. In this sense a therapy session is like a transitional object; the object/session is controlled in somewhat magical fashion entirely by its owner while the rest of the world may be seen as operating in its own chaotic and unruly fashion. Holding on to the 'baa' or the session can make this tolerable. In the session Angela may fantasise that she has control of me through withdrawing and she can then explore what that means for her and how disappointed and angry she in fact feels.

First steps to autonomy

Holding on to this 'baa' (the structure of the session) each woman began slowly to unravel the entangling strings which prevented her from existing separately. This did not so much mean taking huge risks or exploring exciting new emotions with me but rather looking precisely and carefully at just how the strings were tied so as to be able to unknot them rather than tie them tighter. This meant looking at the feelings behind the unconscious and desperate clinging to their identification with their mothers. Angela had been able to leave home when she was still in her teens but behind this independence was her mothering of others; in looking at her attempts to control her therapy by mothering me we learned how frightened she was of letting me see her neediness. She was convinced that it would drive me away; that I would seduce her into revealing her vulnerability and then drop her. She felt that she always became more open just before my holidays and that I deliberately organised this; she was also concerned about the future of the WTC and the possibility of me getting a different job. How could she know that I wouldn't suddenly dump her? When she withdrew and started missing sessions just before I went on holiday we were able to look at the way in which she protected herself from intimacy and she began to feel strongly what it was that she wanted from her relationships. Instead of conducting her relationships as a sort of obstacle course she could contemplate acknowledging her need for closeness. In our session one day I became aware of a moment where the feeling between us was intense and I felt the tears coming to my eyes as if she had allowed us to have contact; the next minute she was rattling on and I had to pull her back and point out what it was that she was rushing away from.

Giving up her identity as an ill person was excruciating for Evelyn. She felt horribly alone and she blamed me. She felt that I had ruined her life by suggesting to her that she might not need to spend the rest of it on metaphorical crutches. The point was not that I had made any suggestions to her but that she was beginning to feel her fury at her mother for not having been available to her outside of the 'nurse' role and she was terrified by the different sort of dependent relationship she was establishing with me.

Mary was perhaps the one who was most straightforwardly overwhelmed by despair when she began to become aware of the gap between her fantasised identification with her mother and the reality of her distance from her. She felt both totally dependent on me and totally unable to get anything from me. For a long time it felt as though there was no sense of the sessions as being 'transitional'; this was reality. I think that the depth of Mary's despair came from the extremity of her early life. For her my incapacity to give her anything was real and my role was to hold on to my sense that however hard she pushed me I still knew that I did in fact have something to offer her even if it wasn't exactly what she wanted.

Rage – attacking the object

One very important way of recognising that another person exists separately is to be able to see that they can survive an attack; in fantasy the child believes that its rage is so powerful that it can destroy the other. Thus to see that however powerful the internal experience of rage may be, the external effects are not commensurate, is an important step both towards losing fantasies of omnipotence and destruction towards acknowledging the experience of real power that the woman may now, as an adult, have in the world.

Mary had particular difficulty in examining her destructive feelings towards me. She felt locked in despair and could not let herself acknowledge her desire to attack me. This was partly because she could not bear to contemplate being left alone with her hopelessness and despair and this in turn combined with her fantasy that she could annihilate me, just as she had driven her mother mad. To recognise that she could not destroy me would be to see the limitations of her power and to face the fact that her mother's craziness was outside her control. For a long time she tested out my capacity to tolerate her despair and hoped against hope for some sort of rescue. Eventually she recognised that there was no escape route and got some glimmerings of the possibility of being able to get something from me. This in turn allowed her to begin to hate me. The process was extremely slow and was tempered with her getting a job which was very obviously doing good for others; she hated the job but she seemed to need it in order to prove her value to me and to others.

Angela too felt that she could not attack me; how could she attack the weak and helpless mother? Behind this was the fear that if she did let her rage loose in the sessions there was no knowing what it would do to me or where it would stop. One day the woman in the next room to us was shouting at her therapist so loudly that we could hear her clearly and Angela felt this confirmed her fear that the WTC, and I in particular, could not contain her rage. Recognising that this was her fantasy not only allowed her to dare to attack me but also put her in touch with the painful reality of the limitations of her power and some very sad and tearful sessions followed.

For Evelyn, as we have seen, her rage emerged at the point at which she began to give up her identity as a sick person. Acknowledging that she could relate person to person was in the first instance completely tied up with her attack on me.

Play

A person who is not psychologically separate cannot play, for playing involves moving from the fantasy world (in which we can dream up magic islands, terrible ogres and good fairies) to the world of reality in which we move freely, daring to try things out and being able to see what happens. Culturally this is not a recognised part of women's role. Women's creativity has often been harnessed in the service of others in order to decorate ourselves to please others.

Though Evelyn's life when she first came to therapy appeared to include many leisure activities, she was quite unable to play. Her striking appearance and the way she engaged in relationships were entirely directed towards getting an appropriate response from others. As she began to attack me she began to feel more freedom in the sessions and could allow herself to roam from one phrase to the next – free associating in an almost classical sense. Later she used her sessions to explore her fears of playing intellectually in her life outside. She discovered herself to be far more intellectually capable than she had ever imagined.

With Mary I first recognised that playing (or rather not playing) was an issue when I realised the difference in my sessions with her from the 'style' I had with other clients. Normally once the client is well established in therapy I do not ask many questions and try not to interrupt the free flow of their associations. With Mary I was still having to prompt her to speak, encouraging her to fill out her remarks. I pointed this out to her and we realised that I was unconsciously picking up on her need to feel directed all the time in order to feel safe. After this we were able to look at her anxieties about playing more freely.

Angela was always too concerned about me and my responses to be able to play. However she did have her own particular stilted form of a game and it was through this that she was able to learn to play more freely. We realised that by being often late for a session or by missing one, she was running away from me, and then waiting for me to run after her. She was quite disappointed when I did not jump to her bait and show her that I cared for her by getting angry, demanding her presence, or questioning her closely as to where she had been when she missed a session. This she interpreted as my not caring. We connected this to the way in which her mother was always avidly interested in what she did, ate or wore. This had been her mother's version of attending to Angela's needs. Very slowly Angela began to experience me in the sessions as a caring person who would watch her spontaneous play rather than seeing my low level of intervention as a sign of neglect.

Autonomy; envy and competition

As a woman begins to feel that her life is changing and that she is able to have a sense of direction stemming from herself she encounters an apparently huge hurdle in the therapy. What if she competes with me and even does better than me? Will I envy her and will I try to stop her? As a woman how can she have more than another woman? We might translate this as a mother's prescription that her daughter follow in her footsteps and stay a second-class citizen in a male world. It is here that I see most clearly the way in which (as Mitchell reminded us, see p.96) women's development is always experienced within the context of patriarchy. If we lose this thread as therapists we cannot do justice to our clients as they move towards leaving therapy.

Therapy groups often provide the clearest reflection of culturally influenced unconscious structures. In a women's group there is often great fear of exciting another's envy. A woman returning from an exciting conference abroad can only talk about her anxieties for fear of how others will feel about her success. Differences in the amount that each woman pays to attend the group are ignored. The strength of the group appears to lie in their identification through distress and oppression. This identification is what they are afraid they will have to give up if they do manage to feel better. They do not know how they will get support and nurturance if they are strong and separate.

These issues came up for Angela, Mary and Evelyn. Angela made real improvements in her standard of living and her work situation but she persisted in seeing herself as an underdog. She could not allow herself to relax into enjoying her relationships or some of the fruits of the money she earned. In therapy she seemed to be going around in miserable circles. She complained bitterly about the money she was wasting on therapy. Since we have an income-related sliding scale at the WTC she was by this point paying quite a high fee and she was constantly reminding me that if she didn't have to pay for therapy she could have been buying a new flat. Then we began to see that in fact we were stuck in a 'vicious' circle. If Angela allowed herself to enjoy her life more she would begin to feel that she no longer needed therapy; she could only have a relationship with me if she was distressed or if she was looking after me. Moreover if she did feel ready to leave therapy she would be able to use her money to buy herself something that she wanted instead of spending it on therapy, which she saw as a legacy of her deprived background. Linking this to her relationship with her mother it seemed that if she had all kinds of things that her mother had never had, then the tie between them would be severed. She would feel alone in the world. Evelyn was also convinced that she would lose her relationship with her mother if she was too successful; however her fear was of her mother's envy and competitiveness. She constantly compared herself with me. Who earned more money? Who had a better degree? Did I feel stuck in my job as a therapist at the WTC? Did I ride a bicycle because I couldn't afford a car or because I was a health freak? When Mary started to have similar thoughts her reaction was to want to escape from therapy.

My role in this was to understand how frightening it was for each woman to contemplate overtaking her mother and thus really acknowledging her separation. This would mean a last stage in becoming conscious of what her mother had not given and of each woman's desire to attack and punish her for not having done so. At this point it was essential not to give up the therapy relationship. Each woman needed to stop being the carer and the underdog and to experience her own strength. Along with this came her awareness of her envy, competitiveness and desire to attack me. We struggled to understand this and to see that it was not inconsistent with wanting to be close to me. We tried to acknowledge each woman's capacity to be a strong person, who could also at times feel distressed and in need of support and understanding.

Conclusion

I began by drawing an analogy between the beginning of the autonomous women's movement and the process of separation at a psychological level. This is not to psychologise social and political issues but rather to see if the one can illuminate the other.

I have used my own experience of psychotherapy with women to illustrate my argument that women can be helped through the therapy relationship to become psychologically separate; yet this is likely to have social implications if we recognise that traditional women's roles are often linked to a lack of psychological separation. Does this mean that the end of psychological separation. Does this mean that the end product of the therapy is likely to be a woman who feels ill at ease within society? Similarly, in the early days of the WTC, people used to ask us 'Will this therapy you are offering lead to broken marriages?'

The link is of course far more complex, as I have tried to suggest. Social changes, which in turn are the result of political struggle, affect the possibilities that are open to women. This includes the availability of therapy for at least some women. Already we are talking about a society in which it is possible to question traditional female roles; in which a woman can choose to have a heterosexual relationship and not have children. The choices women make may be at variance with what is internally acceptable. In choosing not to have children a woman also gives up the unconscious solution (or pseudo-solution) to her difficulty in separating from her mother: namely to reproduce the non-separated relationship. Or a woman may simply feel that she has a right to have more joy and excitement in her life than she saw her mother having. Social change and expectations lead women to seek new ways of resolving their inner conflicts. In turn, the woman who through therapy becomes more psychologically separate may find herself facing new struggles in her everyday life.

She may find that she is less able or willing to defer in what she wants to the interests of others and is therefore less pleasing to men, to her family and to her colleagues. Others may find her threatening. She herself may feel frightened by the way she responds. One woman felt that it was my fault, as her therapist, that she now felt herself to be so alone in the world and to be so relatively unprotected. Individual solutions are not sufficient. Just as in the early days of the women's movement women gained strength through groups which concentrated on their common experience, so now there is a need for those women who are beginning to experience themselves as psychologically separate to struggle for social institutions which validate and allow their difference. At the WTC we have been and still are engaged in precisely this struggle. Can we allow each other to be different, and yet co-operate and support each other?

I am also making a point about psychotherapy. Namely, that in understanding the social context in which our clients were brought up and now live, we are better able to perceive differently the nature of their internal world. This is not saying that there is a precise one-to-one correspondence between the two realms. But it is asserting the view that there is a relationship between the nature of unconscious fantasy and the social world.

In the process of separating, differences may be emphasised in ways that appear divisive and destructive; similarities and continuities may temporarily need to be put aside in the interest of establishing difference. Just because women have found differentiation so difficult psychologically and because there has been no model of positive relationships between differentiated women, divisions have seemed particularly rigid. This has been true in some sections of the women's movement. It has also been true of feminists who are therapists. We have sometimes failed to see the continuity between our work and that of our psychoanalytic predecessors. It has therefore been my concern to illustrate the continuity between Winnicott's writings and feminist work on the mother—daughter relationship.

Acknowledgments

When we run a workshop on 'separation' at the WTC weekend course it is not very popular. Separation has been a difficult subject for me to face and write about. In the long-drawn-out process of freeing myself to write this chapter I was helped by my therapy group at the Institute of Group Analysis, by living through different phases of separation with my daughters, Sarah, Emma and Rosie and by sharing the separation/mourning for our mother with my sister, Eva.

I am also grateful to my clients who time and again led me back to the ideas I have written about.

Sheila Ernst

Notes

1.　Charles Bernheimer and Claire Kahane (eds), *In Dora's Case*, Virago, London 1985.
2.　C. Rycroft, *Dictionary of Psychoanalysis*, Penguin, Harmondsworth, 1972, p.68.
3.　D.W. Winnicott, 'The theory of the parent—infant relationship', 1960, in *The Maturational Processes and the Facilitating Environment*, Hogarth Press, London, 1965, pp.37-56.
4.　Sheila Rowbotham, *Women's Consciousness, Man's World*, Penguin, Harmondsworth, 1973, p.28.
5.　ibid., p.27.
6.　Marsha Rowe (ed.), *Spare Rib Reader*, Penguin, Harmondsworth, 1982, p.16.
7.　Rowbotham, *Women's Consciousness, Man's World*, p.30.
8.　ibid.
9.　Malcolm Pines, 'Reflections on mirroring', *Group Analysis*, XV (2), supplement, 1982.
10.　J. Vellacott, 'Ambivalence in early motherhood', unpublished paper, p.34.
11.　Rowbotham, *Women's Consciousness, Man's World*, p.32.
12.　ibid., p.35.
13.　Paul Scott, *The Jewel in the Crown*, Panther, London, 1984, p.352.
14.　Sara Davidson, *Loose Change*, Fontana, London, 1978.
15.　Marge Piercy, *Small Changes*, Fawcett Crest, New York, 1973.
16.　Doris Lessing, *The Golden Notebook*, Granada, London, 1973.
17.　Kate Millett, *Sita,* Virago, London, 1977.
18.　D.W. Winnicott, 'The location of cultural experience' in *Playing and Reality*, Penguin, Harmondsworth, 1974, p.116.
19.　P. Adams, 'Mothering', *M/F*, 1983, pp.41-51.
20.　Winnicott, 'The theory of the parent—infant relationship', p.53.
21.　ibid.
22.　Winnicott, 'Primary maternal preoccupation' in *Through Paediatrics to Psychoanalysis*, Hogarth Press, London, 1982, pp.300-305.
23.　Ann Oakley, *From Here to Maternity*, Penguin, Harmondsworth, 1981.
24.　Winnicott, 'Primary maternal preoccupation', p.302.

Can a daughter be a woman? 115

25. Nancy Chodorow, *The Reproduction of Mothering*, University of California Press, Berkeley, Cal., 1978.
26. Winnicott, 'Creativity and its origins' in *Playing and Reality*.
27. M. Davis and D. Wallbridge, *Boundary and Space*, Karnac, London, 1981. (See section 10, 'Dependence and domination', pp.131-41.)
28. Winnicott, 'Mirror role of mother and family' in *Playing and Reality*, pp.132-3.
29. ibid.
30. Winnicott, 'The theory of the parent–infant relationship', p.51.
31. Marilyn Lawrence, *The Anorexic Experience*, The Women's Press, London, 1984.
32. Margaret S. Mahler, Fred Pine and Anni Bergman, *The Psychological Birth of the Human Infant*, Basic Books, New York, 1975.
33. Winnicott, 'Transitional objects and phenomena' in *Playing and Reality*.
34. ibid., p.5.
35. Winnicott, 'Playing: a theoretical statement' in *Playing and Reality*, p.55.
36. Sigmund Freud, quoted in Nancy Chodorow, *The Reproduction of Mothering*, p.92.
37. Juliet Mitchell, 'Freud and Lacan: psychoanalytic theories of sexual difference' in *Women: the longest revolution*, Virago, London, 1984, p.252.
38. Other psychoanalysts in this broad tradition drawn on in this book include W. Bion, D. Fairbairn, H. Guntrip and M. Klein.
39. Mitchell, 'Freud and Lacan' in *Women: the longest revolution*, p.274.
40. Chodorow, op. cit, p.103.
41. ibid.
42. ibid., p.169.
43. Luise Eichenbaum and Susie Orbach, *Outside In ... Inside Out*, Penguin, Harmondsworth, 1982.
44. J. Flax, 'The conflict between nurturance and autonomy in mother/daughter relations within feminism', *Women and Mental Health*, eds Elizabeth Howell and Marjorie Bayes, Basic Books, New York, 1981.
45. J. Ryan, 'Psychoanalysis and women loving women' in S. Cartledge and J. Ryan (eds), *Sex and Love*, The Women's Press, London, 1983, p.205.

46. D. Pines, 'Skin communication: Early skin disorders and their effect on transference and counter transference' *Int. J. Psychoanal.* (1980), 61 pt. III, pp.315-23.
47. ibid.
48. R. Coward, *Female Desire*, Paladin, London, 1984.
49. Mitchell, *Women: the longest revolution*, p.273.
50. ibid.
51. ibid., p.274.
52. Janet Sayers, 'Psychoanalysis and Personal Politics,' *Feminist Review*, 10, 1982, pp.91-5.
53. V. Jelenevsky Seidler, 'Trusting ourselves: Marxism, human needs and sexual politics' in Simon Clark, Terry Lovell, Kevin McDonnell, Kevin Robin and V. Jelenevsky Seidler, *One Dimensional Marxism* Allison Busby, London, 1980, p.114.
54. L. Segal, 'Sexual uncertainty or why the clitoris is not enough', in S. Cartledge and J. Ryan (eds), *Sex and Love*.

5
Casting the evil eye – women and envy

Women do not wish to become men, but want to detach themselves from the mother, and become complete autonomous *women*.

When I admire someone I want to be them. When I realise I can't become them, envy sets in and I start to tear them to bits.[1]

Introduction

It has traditionally been assumed within our culture that women have a strong streak of covert envy, spite and malice that emerges in a particularly virulent form with other members of their own sex. Feminists, on the other hand, have often expressed the hope that envious and competitive feelings would prove to be a product of capitalism and patriarchy, and would become less intense or even disappear completely as women developed more open and co-operative relationships with each other. This hope has, however, frequently been undermined by the powerful and unconscious nature of envious feelings. In this chapter, I concentrate on the complex dynamics of envy between women. While I recognise the strength of envy between the sexes, I do not focus on women's envy of men. I explore instead the way in which all envy originates within the infant's earliest and most fundamental relationship, which is usually with the mother,[2] and the specific effects of mother–daughter envy on the girl's developing sense of herself.

In recent years there has been a change in women's role and expectations, and feminism itself has been highly influential in increasing our sense of confidence and self-value. Some women have more freedom to develop, but new pressures have also been created. As we struggle to establish ourselves in unfamiliar territories we may find ourselves competing with other women more intensely and in different areas of our lives. Traditionally, women have compared their looks, their relationships with men, and their capacities as mothers. Now, in addition, we may compare our work and financial status, and perhaps even our abilities to project a strong feminist image. It seems that, yet again, we have to acknowledge that we are dealing with a problem that is not merely external. An awareness of the effects of unconscious envy on our ability to learn, create, and sustain close loving relationships forces us to acknowledge that we have to struggle not just with oppressive outer realities but also with the existence of an internal world where feelings and fantasies may contradict our conscious beliefs and aspirations.

Jealousy and competition are sometimes discussed by feminists, but envy has received very little attention. This silence may reflect a desire to emphasise feelings of sisterhood and solidarity, but it also mirrors the denial of envy which prevails throughout our society. This powerful emotion, the 'evil eye' of folklore, is now, and has been historically, hidden and disguised, rarely discussed and little understood.

The reluctance even to name envy is reflected in the common habit of confusing it with jealousy when, in fact, the two emotions are quite different. Envy is described in Webster's Dictionary as 'chagrin or discontent at the excellence or good fortune of another'. Jealousy is the fear that a rival will take something away, usually the affections of a third person. The crucial difference is that envy occurs between two people, whereas jealousy involves real or imagined rivalry or competition among at least three people. Envy is, then, a feeling that arises early in an infant's development, while she is still preoccupied with dyadic relationships, whereas jealousy, competition and rivalry, which are all based on and closely related to envy, arise once the child becomes aware of triangular and interconnected networks of relationships within and outside the family. So competition, like jealousy, of which it is a component, does not simply involve covetous and destructive feelings and fantasies about something possessed by another. The child is no longer quite so helpless; she can now compete, or imagine herself competing, with others to win whatever she perceives as desirable. So, I might envy another woman's exciting job. If she seemed to be replacing me in the affections of a close friend, I might feel jealous and competitive. In order to get myself a job like hers, I might well have to enter into actual competition with a number of other people.

But why exactly has envy, of all the emotions, been so strongly denied, concealed, and avoided? It was listed as one of the seven deadly sins by the mediaeval Church and described by Chaucer as the worst of all sins.[3] In Dante's *Inferno* the envious were accorded the most excruciating torture – their eyelids were sewn together.[4] Envy involves the fantasy of possessing what one needs but does not have and is therefore a desperate attempt to protect the self from a recognition of painful feelings of personal inadequacy, humiliation or lack, rather than a real attempt to acquire whatever is desired. Melanie Klein comes closest to capturing the intensely disturbing nature of envy in her essay 'Envy and gratitude', where she describes envy as being an attack on love and creativity; the object of love and admiration, originally the mother, is damaged or destroyed, in fantasy, if not in reality. She believes envy to be a purely destructive emotion, the angry desire to spoil, rob or poison that which is most needed, the source of life itself. She quotes Chaucer, in *The Parson's Tale*, 'It is certain that envy is the worst sin that is; for all other sins are sins only against one virtue, whereas envy is against all virtue and against all goodness.'[5] Klein points out that there is a much more sympathetic social attitude towards jealousy than envy. In some countries jealousy can actually be used as a mitigating factor in sentencing for murder. This she attributes to a universal sense that jealousy, unlike envy, implies the existence of love, and an impulse to preserve it. Jealousy may reflect possessiveness, insecurity and vanity, as much as any loving concern, but nevertheless it is generally thought of as a much more presentable if not always a creditable feeling. We can allow ourselves to remain conscious of our jealousy, whereas we are likely to be unconscious of our envy. Envy is too painful for conscious awareness; as adults we cannot tolerate the powerful and confusing infantile feelings of need, helplessness and destructiveness with which it is associated. The infant who has been exposed to unbearable early experiences of deprivation or humiliation develops a deep-rooted sense of personal inadequacy which will cause her, as she grows older, continually to compare herself enviously with others. Inextricably linked as it is with these feelings of deep personal inadequacy, and with the desire to steal or spoil whatever is most needed and admired, envy, while it remains unconscious, will have an acutely destructive effect on the self and on relationships with others. But if feelings of envy, inferiority and rage can be consciously acknowledged and accepted, the envious person can perhaps learn and develop through emulating those she admires.

In recent years there has been much discussion amongst feminists and socialists about the desirability of eradicating competitiveness. In fact it is impossible to imagine this happening in any society, even when the political organisation emphasises equality and co-operation. It has been pointed out that there is a word for envy in almost every language,[6] and rivalry seems inherent in childhood experience. The first real inequality for all of us is the experience of being small, powerless and utterly dependent on the adults around us. Inevitably, there will be other demands on the mother's attention. These inequities and the painful necessity of sharing love give rise to feelings of inadequacy, frustration, humiliation, rage, jealousy and rivalry.

If she can be helped to struggle with difficulties rather than to accommodate to them, the child's developing personality will be strengthened. Her parents' capacities to give her love and protection while, at the same time, helping her tolerate internal conflicts, will be influenced by their own childhood experiences. The child's way of negotiating these fundamental experiences of inequality with parents and siblings, and the help she is given, will lay the basis for her capacity to struggle with the whole range of real material inequities she will encounter in later life, such as those of age, health, sex, class and race. If she has been helped to deal with childhood rivalries, squabbles and rows, and has learned to persevere in attempting to get what she wants, to hold her own, but also to share, she will have had some preparation for the inevitable difficulties of adulthood. So an ability to recognise and value our own needs and desires, and to compete when necessary, may derive from a sense of inner strength, unlike envy which springs from feelings of inadequacy. For someone who cannot compete at all, everyday possibilities are seriously restricted.

Boys and girls are equally likely to be exposed to experiences that give rise to feelings of pain, humiliation, inferiority, envy and hostility, but these emotions will later be dealt with internally and expressd externally in different ways. Girls, who tend to remain more in touch with internal processes, and who tend to be receptive, nurturing and intuitive, are likely to be more aware of feelings of lack, inadequacy and envy, while denying any associated aggression. Boys, whose upbringing restricts their awareness of emotional life, while strengthening pseudo-adult structures which enable them to 'manage' in the external world, will tend to cut off from feelings of vulnerability and inadequacy and use their aggression to compete. They are encouraged to become overtly competitive and fiercely rivalrous. Girls, on the other hand, have few opportunities to fight for what they want openly, and to see that this need not necessarily hurt others or have a detrimental effect on themselves. They are likely to develop an intense fear of competition, learning to limit their expectations and desires, to get what they want by indirect means, to experience pleasure and success vicariously, through identification with partners or children. Whereas the male stereotype is of blatant rivalry – boasting, showing off, telling anecdotes designed to impress, women are more likely to hesitate, deprecate, hide their strengths and play down their assets.

The meaning of terms like 'personal achievement' and 'success' are problematic for many people within our society, but particularly so for women, since prestige and power have traditionally been associated with male activities. Women have to deal not only with current everyday realities of discrimination, but also with the personal and political implications of accepting or rejecting traditional notions of success and fulfilment and, on a psychological level, with their own internalised feelings and fantasies, which may conflict with conscious desires and expectations.

In this chapter I focus on the dynamics of envy between women, particularly within the therapy relationship. I argue that whilst we can learn much from existing psychoanalytic ideas about envy, these need supplementing with a feminist understanding of women's social position and psychological development. This I do by looking first in some detail at the specific experiences of several women, and then by placing these individual accounts within a more generalised framework concerning the impact of gender.

In describing the way envy manifests itself, and its effects on women's lives, I shall draw mainly on my experience as a group and individual psychotherapist, but also on accounts that women have given me of their relationships.[7]

The experience of envy – accounts by women

The following discussion about envy in a psychodynamically orientated women's therapy group illustrates the very different ways the group members expressed this feeling and defended themselves from consciously experiencing it. One woman admitted that she dreaded being singled out for praise, as she had been in her dance class that morning. It gradually emerged that she had always feared getting special attention from the group therapist since she imagined that this would 'spoil' her relationships with the other women, who might then resent her. It was pointed out to her by another group member that she habitually denigrated those aspects of her life that might arouse envy in others. In a group where several of the other women had unsatisfactory sexual relationships and where most were unemployed or unhappy with their working lives, she took care not to dwell on the fact that her long marriage had always been sexually passionate and that she had been highly successful in the career she had pursued until her first child was born. Instead, she emphasised the aspects of her sexual and emotional life that were problematic, and criticised her previous work for personal and political reasons. The woman who dreaded being praised then began to talk about the way she had feared the envy and retaliation of her fragile and sickly sister. Using a childhood analogy, she said to the group, 'I'll make quite sure you don't want my teddy bear.' Another woman in the group said that she couldn't understand this, since she herself devoted enormous effort to making other people envy her. She was aware that she boasted about the good things in her life and didn't mention the difficulties. She usually painted a glorious picture of her family life, and it had taken her months to admit the problems that had brought her to the group. 'I want you to want my teddy bear', she said. A third woman said that she was highly competitive. 'I always want everything everyone else has, and I try to get it. I want the group's attention all the time, and I want to be group therapist. I want you to admire me. I want your teddy bear and I also want you to want mine.' Another woman who usually found it hard to talk about herself, said that she habitually idealised the lives of other women in the group. 'I always think other people's teddy bears must be better than mine. I envy you all the time, but I can't imagine anyone envying me.' The envious person may protect herself against awareness of her own feelings by projecting them into other people, whom she then experiences as envious and destructive. She will then be afraid to reveal anything admirable in herself, lest they spoil it in some way as, unconsciously, she feels she would do if she were in their shoes.

In working individually with women, it becomes apparent how deeply envy can affect each woman's sense of herself, her ability to be creative and to sustain close relationships.

Jenny

Jenny came to therapy feeling desperately miserable, anxious, and empty inside. She'd worked in offices and shops after leaving school, and was now unemployed. Initially I found her touchingly open and vulnerable, but I soon realised that building a relationship with her would be a painfully slow and frustrating process. She sat through her sessions in a terrified silence, allowing herself to absorb nothing beneficial from me. Her experience was of losing, or feeling that she destroyed, anything she valued. Whenever she made a positive move in her life she would sabotage it immediately; after a helpful session she would miss the next. She felt that if she was getting too close to me she must move away again quickly, in case her presence damaged me or made me ill.

Jenny related her deep feelings of loneliness and inadequacy to a series of separations in early childhood from her mother, who had frequently been ill. With her parents she had felt in various ways both envied and envious, inadequate and deprived, yet special and lucky. She lived in the shadow of her mother, whose extrovert personality she admired and envied. As Jenny's parents' marriage became increasingly strained, she felt that her mother, who was now very unhappy, envied and resented her ability to gain her father's attention. Jenny developed a deprecating manner and a habit of denigrating anything she had at home and at school, fearing particularly that she would lose her mother's love if she shone in the eyes of the world.

For a long time in therapy Jenny presented herself to me as entirely bereft of assets and resources, only gradually showing me glimpses of her strengths, fearing that if I was aware of them I would undermine her with envious or critical comments, or reject her as too fortunate to need my help. At the same time she envied and idealised me as she had her mother, endowing me in her fantasies with the qualities and lifestyle she herself wanted.

When Jenny was fifteen her father left the family and her mother's physical health deteriorated drastically. As Jenny's therapy progressed, it became clear that she felt unconsciously deeply guilty about these occurrences, fearing that she'd damaged her mother through her demands for attention and her temper tantrums, and exacerbated the rift between her parents through occasional moments of closeness with her emotionally distant father. Everyday childhood competition had proved unsafe for Jenny. Her rival had not survived the battle intact. Her mother, whose life was becoming increasingly lonely and restricted, appeared to begrudge Jenny her new-found popularity and seemed to panic at her moves towards independence. Both made desperate demands for support and understanding, but were totally unable to provide it for each other. Unconsciously, Jenny felt unable to continue to grow up and to make a fulfilling adult life for herself. It seemed that womanhood could only be achieved at her mother's expense.

Envy is often associated with a lack of self-worth and an insecure, tenuous or fragmented sense of self. As a result of intolerable experiences of deprivation and loneliness during her early childhood separations from her mother, Jenny had developed strong doubts about her own goodness and worth. She envied and resented her mother's power to give and withhold love from her, and began constantly to compare herself unfavourably with other people around her. Having been unable, through her early relationship with her mother, to develop a sense of internal harmony, Jenny's feelings of envy and resentment were later exacerbated by an awareness of her mother's admiration, envy and hostility towards her. Jenny's fear that she would destroy, through her envy and aggression, anything she took inside herself made it difficult for her to use therapy or any other learning situation to develop a stronger, more integrated sense of herself. She had a history of disappointments and failures, and each new setback further undermined her confidence in herself as a competent and creative person. In these characteristics she corresponds to Melanie Klein's description of people whose internal good object, their sense of self as lovable and valuable, is very precariously established.[8] Like them, Jenny was fearful and anxious that her sense of self would be spoiled or destroyed by her own or other people's competitive and envious feelings, and therefore avoided competition and success.

Pauline

Pauline's early sessions consisted of a non-stop litany of major and minor disasters. Her 'busyness' prevented anyone getting close to her and although she was constantly surrounded by people, her relationships seemed devoid of intimacy or enjoyment. It was a shock to me when, some time later, I realised how fortunate and successful Pauline might have seemed, if I had been shown only the external details of her life. She described an early family atmosphere of guilt, envy and deprivation. Her needs had always seemed secondary to those of her mother. At school and with her peers she was praised and valued; but at home everything she achieved was either taken for granted or disparaged. Now, as an adult, she had internalised the capacity to destroy her own sense of herself as capable, attractive or successful by continually tormenting herself over minor and often imaginary failures. Pauline associated these internal voices with a fear of her parents' envy and a series of prohibitions against taking pride in and enjoying her talents and good fortune. She was consumed with unconscious guilt about having succeeded not only in traditional female terms, but also in the male world of work, although consciously she felt she had a perfect right to live a full life. She had already surpassed her father, who was, like her, an accountant, and felt that he resented this bitterly.

But Pauline's most intense conflicts and fears were focused around the possibility of gaining a way of life that could clearly be seen to be different from, and more fulfilling than, her mother's, and of having confidence in her own feelings and judgments. Pauline had internalised a prohibition about enjoying sexuality or projecting herself as feminine if she wanted herself to be taken seriously as a person. While she desperately wanted to feel independent from her mother, a whole person in her own right, she feared that she would hurt or damage her mother, or lose her love through incurring her envy and retaliation.

In her therapy, Pauline unconsciously reproduced with me the pattern of her relationship with her mother and her friendships with women. Initially, she felt overwhelmed by misery and totally dependent on my help. I became for her an entirely idealised figure, the possessor of all emotional riches. She felt that, through listening to her, and helping her to understand her unconscious fantasies and to contain and accept her own feelings and needs, I was giving her, as an adult, some of the experiences she had lacked in her early relationship with her mother. She began to envy the perfect image she had created of me, and to resent my ability to help her; but initially her idealisation of me and her denigration of herself also protected her against awareness of these feelings. Gradually she began to make changes in her life. Her relationships deepened as she became aware of a wider range of feelings, and she began to relax some of her internal prohibitions against pleasure. She began to acknowledge her own resources, saying, 'My parents must have given me something, since I've been successful.'

However, she was also making it clear, despite desperate struggles not to acknowledge it, that her image of me had changed drastically. She had begun to experience me as she had her mother, as overwhelmingly envious, controlling and withholding. This may well have reflected the internalised experience of a mother who was in reality envious and begrudging, but this image was intensified by projections of her own unconscious envy and hostility. Although she had been previously unaware of it, she had felt herself to be almost totally merged with me, psychologically, as she still was with her mother. Now, as she struggled to separate herself from me and from her internalised persecuting mother-image, she experienced both her desire for independence and her rage and envy as overwhelmingly dangerous for all of us.

The extent to which Pauline remained, in the early part of her therapy, unaware of her desire to tear me down off the pedestal she'd put me on, trample all over me and perhaps put herself in my place, and her acute difficulties in accepting those feelings and fantasies later, does of course reflect her socialisation as a woman to deny her aggression. Similarly, the prolonged and intensely painful nature of her struggle to assert herself as an independent, whole woman reflects a complex interrelationship of psychological and socio-political factors. A girl may, as Pauline did, have internalised (alongside a whole set of moral and social prohibitions) a powerful feeling that she should not find a place for herself in a male world, or that if she did, it should only be by renouncing all the external signs of her femaleness. At an unconscious level Pauline also had to cope with her fears about having usurped and damaged her father in his traditional masculine role. Pauline's sense of frustration about not being able to break free of her internalised mother without triumphing over and damaging her, reflects the continued strength and ambivalence of the tie between mother and daughter. Unlike a boy, a girl cannot use biological difference to differentiate herself from her mother. As Janine Chasseguet-Smirgel points out, the girl has nothing the mother doesn't have, and is therefore unable to show her independence clearly. She points out that the woman's apparent desire to have what is usually associated with masculine power, traditionally referred to as 'penis envy' is the symbolic expression of another desire. In fact, 'Women do not wish to become men, but want to detach themselves from the mother and become complete autonomous *women*.'[9]

In the early part of her therapy, Pauline, like many women, used constant self-criticism to distract attention away from her own inner strength and her actual achievements. This devaluation of the self, as Klein points out, serves both as a denial of envy and a punishment for it.[10] In therapy, as elsewhere, it also greatly increases envious feelings towards others.

Some women's personal strengths and good fortune emerge as a series of major 'secrets', revealed only as the therapy progresses. For example, one woman emphasised in her early sessions that her only talent was for attracting men. She couldn't understand why, since she considered herself to be fat and ugly and felt persecuted by their attentions. My view of her changed dramatically when one day she let slip a clue to the fact that, all through her educational and working life, she had shown herself to be exceptionally capable and responsible. It transpired that what she had actually portrayed as a brief, desultory, yet painful foray into social work had actually been a highly successful short career, punctuated by meteorically fast leaps up the promotion ladder. It gradually became clear that presenting herself as an entirely resourceless victim enabled this woman to enlist sympathy and support for her vulnerabilities from me and other people, without arousing the envy she feared if she demonstrated her strengths.

Envy consists of a combination of intensely contradictory emotions. The envious person feels admiration, inadequacy, rage, hostility, guilt, and the desire to spoil, steal, or triumph over. The intense pain and anxiety involved creates a distance between the envious person and those she envies. So Pauline's fears that she would damage any potentially nurturing figure, as she felt she had damaged her mother, made it difficult for her to allow close emotional contact with me in therapy. Another client described similar fears. 'When I admire someone I want to be them. When I realise I can't become them, envy sets in and I start to tear them to bits.' This woman maintained a distance from me by what she described as a 'secret armoury' of contemptuous criticism, so avoiding both intimacy and dependency and any attendant feelings of admiration, inadequacy, envy and hostility. The tendency to spoil and devalue whatever is envied is both an expression of envy and a defence against it, since once the coveted attributes are destroyed, in fantasy or reality, they can no longer arouse the same painful feelings. The very envious person who assumes an air of superiority and silently criticises the person she envies, is not only disowning her own envy but may, unconsciously, be attempting to arouse similar feelings of envy, discomfort and inadequacy in the person she admires. She would not then be experiencing her envy; but would be trying, unconsciously, to make the other person bear her own intolerable feelings.

Because it is linked with feelings of inferiority, envy inhibits the creation of all relationships where the individual can learn, grow or change. This affects relationships with teachers or therapists (as in Pauline's therapy). Another woman, describing her difficulties in learning, said, 'I've got to find my own way, stay in control. To allow anyone to help me means I'll lose myself, get taken over.' Because of her dislike of hierarchies, this envious woman gravitated towards leaderless, self-help therapy groups. But, since envy also impedes the creation of equal and openly co-operative relationships with peers, she could not allow herself to be open and vulnerable enough to change and develop within this setting, either. Her behaviour was typical of that shown by very envious people in groups of all kinds. She held herself aloof, an air of silent superiority belying her deep-rooted fear of being discovered to be inferior to others.

Joan and Olivia

The following account illustrates the way that an idealised closeness between women friends can break down into envy and aggressive competitiveness.

Joan and Olivia had been close friends for nearly three years. Joan described the early part of their friendship as having a

charmed quality – dramatic and intense – as if we had a magic circle around us that excluded other people. Striding into any social gathering with Olivia I felt I could take the world on . . . march in and kick the door down. When I feel passionately about someone, I almost want to be that person, and that's how I felt about Olivia. We seemed to let down psychological barriers with each other through talking that I'd only ever let down with other people if I had sex with them.

But it seems that when I tell someone else all about me, identity confusions arise. I stop knowing where I end and the other person begins. I wanted Olivia's approval so desperately that I began to lose track of why I was doing things. I finally realised that I needed to find myself again. But then we started to argue really bitterly. I can see now that we were always competitive.

But when we were close we operated as a kind of unit. It was OK for her to be wonderful because I felt I basked in her reflected glory. When we separated we both lost out. We'd never criticised each other before, but then we had to continually undermine what the other had in order to prove that we were better. I began to see her as a kind of monster. I felt I'd let Olivia step right over my psychological boundaries. When she wore one of my dresses without asking, it was as if she'd got right into my skin, as if she was about to take me over completely. With Dave, I also feel competitive, but it's different. I realise I can never become him and he can't become me. The sexual differences between us mean that we can only merge up to a point.

Joan notes that she feels a similar sense of being ambivalently 'stuck' in relation to her mother, a strong woman, who had found few outlets for her creative energies. 'My mother seemed, when I was a child, to project a lot of her unhappiness and frustration on to me – as if I was a part of her that stopped her doing things. Now I feel it's as if she's saying to me, "You're not OK. You're not what I want you to be. Hang on to me."' In order to develop a sense of who she is, the baby needs to look at the mother's face and to feel that she herself is being reflected there, that she has been seen by the mother, so she exists. Joan does not seem to have seen a clear reflection of herself in her mother's face. Instead she saw either her mother's frustration, her expectations for her daughter, or her envy for that imagined future. Joan grew up feeling that there was some deep vulnerability in her that she must keep hidden. She envied those who seemed to have a stronger sense of who they were and what they wanted to do. Through her friendship with Olivia, Joan unconsciously attempted to fulfil some of the needs that her mother had been unable to meet.

Without being aware of it, both women had hoped that, through returning to an infantile state of unity with each other, they could emerge with a stronger sense of self. In fact, the friendship had broken down under the strain of these unspoken desires, into resentment, envy and recrimination.

Joan could see that, at one level, her confusion about who she wanted to be was related to the fact that she had grown up in an 'in-between generation. As a working-class woman who received a professional education, I had no role models.' But she came to realise that psychologically she also felt paralysed by a fear of the consequences of having the kind of life her mother had always wanted. 'If I'd got married young, especially to a middle-class man with money, and had children as well as a professional career, I think she'd have been bitterly jealous. I was afraid of losing her love.'

Joan also discusses the effect of having a father who, although physically present, failed to make his presence felt in the family, to take any emotional weight. 'He did try to come in between me and my mother at times, but my mother was much stronger. She always pushed him out again. So the bond was never broken between us, and I could never get away.'

Similarly, in Jenny and Pauline's families, there was no evidence of a third force, another strong adult presence that would, at a certain point, break into the mother–daughter dyad, reclaiming the mother into the world of adult relationships, and giving the daughter the opportunity to experience a different kind of close relationship with an adult. If, as often happens, even when there is a father present in the family, mother and daughter receive no external support in separating psychologically from each other, the already difficult process of differentiation becomes even harder, and the effects of mother–daughter envy are likely to be exacerbated.

Conscious or unconscious attempts to arouse envy in others, idealisation of the envied person and a preoccupation with the fear of being envied are all ways of denying or defending ourselves against our own envy and conflicts about competitiveness. Envy may be aroused in others in various ways. Some women hide their own envy while exaggerating their strengths. Other women enlist sympathy by appearing pathetic, making other people feel angry, envious and deceived when they unexpectedly reveal their hidden resources. While being envied may temporarily compensate for feelings of inadequacy, eventually the person who arouses envy will either be attacked, or lives in fear that she will be. Since idealisation is an attempt to defend the self against awareness of deprivation, rage, or envy, the idealised person may later be experienced as persecuting and hateful (as in Pauline's therapy, or Joan and Olivia's friendship). When this pattern is extreme, it can lead to the creation of a range of relationships that break down rapidly because no one can live up to the idealised expectations.

The women I have described all use ways of expressing and

defending themselves against envy that correspond with prevailing notions of femininity. Envy and hostility, especially when directed towards other women, are usually denied or expressed indirectly. Strengths and achievements tend to be hidden or devalued, while other people are idealised. Each of these women has a tendency to lose a sense of herself and her own feelings within relationships, and to define herself through identifying with others. The mother who lacks a strong sense of her own value, who feels deprived and envious, will be unable to help her daughter to develop a sense of internal harmony and strength. The daughter, who will then feel inadequate and inferior, will be reinforced in her own envious feelings by experiences of envy within the family. The intense fear of envy expressed by many of these women is, then, both a projection of their own unconscious envy and a reflection of their experience of having had a mother who envied her growing daughter.

Psychoanalytic views on envy

Within psychoanalytic literature, there has been strong debate about the nature and origins of envy, although certain ways of describing this emotion have remained quite consistent. Envy has, for instance, generally been associated with wounded narcissism (damage to the sense of psychological well-being) and has been consistently seen as an impediment to change and growth within analysis. However, while some theorists see very early infantile envy and rage as the source of later personality difficulties, others believe that envy results from, and must be preceded by, experiences of pain, deprivation or humiliation. While Freud focused mainly on female penis-envy (a topic which is beyond the scope of this chapter), discussions rapidly broadened to a consideration of envy as a universal human emotion. Whenever he mentioned envy, Freud described it as arising in later infancy, although he saw the roots of the narcissistic hurt, so fundamental to penis-envy, in the baby's early relationship to the mother's breast: 'The reproach against the mother which goes back furthest is that she gave the child too little milk – which is construed against her as lack of love . . . the child's avidity for its earliest nourishment is altogether insatiable, . . . it never gets over the pain of losing its mother's breast.'[11] Abraham and Jones saw envy and (in Jones' case) a particular kind of envious hatred, as developing gradually during childhood through the interaction between environmental and constitutional factors.[12]

In contrast to this, Melanie Klein stated firmly that envy was an inborn drive, closely linked with the death instinct and purely destructive in its aims. Individuals are born, she believes, with 'different constitutional tendencies towards aggression and envy and with varying capacities for love'.[13] These tendencies are, however, accentuated by the infant's experiences within the womb and during birth. The baby feels envy initially in relation to its first love object (which she assumed to be the mother's breast, or its substitute, the feeding bottle) as a response both to satisfaction and deprivation. Envy is aroused by the baby's awareness that the source of love, comfort and nourishment on which she so utterly depends lies outside herself and cannot be controlled. Attributing considerable psychological sophistication to the infant, Klein describes her as assuming that when she is not being fed her mother must be gratifying herself with the magical richness of the 'feeding breast'.

Klein's views on the origins of envy touch on crucial psychoanalytic controversies – debates about whether aggression is inborn or reactive and the extent to which the very young baby experiences itself as separate from other people. Winnicott's views on the origins of envy are in complete opposition to Klein's. In his view the baby is so incapable of surviving on its own that it is meaningless to discuss it as a separate unit, outside its natural context, which he assumes to be the mother–baby couple. Far from being able to see itself as a separate person, the newborn baby lives in a world of undifferentiated sensations, unaware of whether the finger or nipple it sucks belongs to itself or to someone else. He suggests that the baby who feels secure, satisfied and contented will, by and large, exist in a state of pleasurable unity with the mother. For 'this child the breast is the self and the self is the breast. Envy is a term that might become applicable in the experience of a tantalising failure of the breast as something that is'.[14] If she is aware of sources of nourishment and comfort outside herself, then she must be experiencing a quite serious sense of deprivation or lack.

Susie Orbach and Luise Eichenbaum, in their writings on women's psychological development within patriarchy, describe the way that they see feelings of insecurity, unentitlement, abandonment and anger being distorted and converted into competition, envy, guilt and depression, which then lead to further self-condemnation. Like Winnicott, they believe that envy can only arise as a reaction to experiences of pain or frustration.[15]

Joffe, in his 'Critical review of the status of the envy concept', says that babies are not yet psychologically sophisticated enough to feel what he calls envy 'proper', and points out that Klein's account of infantile envy attributes to the baby not only the ability, at birth, to see itself as separate from the mother, but also the capacity to think about the absent mother's motives and intentions. The infant must, he says, not only be able to wish for something it lacks, but also be able to fantasise about what it might be like to possess the desired object, before it can really be capable of envy. He also points out that, since envy is a complex emotional attitude closely related to less sophisticated feeling states, such as possessiveness, it is very difficult, given our lack of really concrete knowledge about early childhood, to delineate an exact point at which envy might arise as a separate and distinct emotion or character trait. He emphasises that envy is always linked not just to aggression and destructive fantasies, but also to love or admiration, and says that experiences that give rise to a deep sense of personal inadequacy, and thence to envy, may occur during all stages of childhood and adolescent development.

In fact, Klein and Joffe are defining envy in different ways. What Klein is describing is the powerful early rage and need of the infant who is unable to control the mother's breast. Her own aggressive and destructive fantasies give rise to intolerable feelings of terror in the infant who fears that she will annihilate both herself and the mother on whom she utterly depends. This feeling is so unbearable that it is made unconscious. While Klein emphasises the primitive destructiveness of unconscious envy, Joffe focuses on a later more complicated character trait which arises because the child, due to actual painful or humiliating experiences, has internalised a feeling of having a 'massive fantasied disability'. Joffe emphasises the links between envy and admiration and the possibility of using envy constructively. Klein refers only briefly to a later form of envy arising at the toddler stage which is based on early envy but also associated with rivalry and jealousy.[16]

I do not agree with Klein that envy is linked with an innate drive towards aggression although obviously, as she points out, the newborn infant has already had important formative experiences. It does seem, however, that the emotional state described by Klein may be the precursor of adult envy, and that these powerful infantile feelings and fantasies continue unconsciously to be associated with the more complicated character trait described by Joffe. We cut ourselves off from conscious awareness of envy and regard it with such universal horror precisely because of this link with feelings of infantile helplessness and with fears of destroying both love and life itself. Once we become conscious of our envy and can integrate it with feelings such as admiration and gratitude, it will lose some of its destructive potential.

In my experience, whenever a client is strongly and consistently envious of others, the reasons for this can be located within her early history. Usually there has been a history of frustration or deprivation in the first years of life. The child who has been unbearably exposed to her own helplessness and vulnerability, who has suffered some significant lack of attention, feels reduced, and therefore compares herself enviously with others. Sometimes envy can be connected with experiences of physical and emotional pain or humiliation in later childhood or adolescence. Often, too, the client comes to recognise that envy has been strongly present between mother and daughter and also between other family members. So, Jenny's difficulties in digesting and assimilating my help during the therapy sessions and her urge to sabotage anything which might potentially be beneficial, may have originated in very primitive aggressive and 'envious' reactions to the deprivations she experienced while separated from her mother as an infant. But both she and Pauline also describe a later, more sophisticated form of envy associated with the desire to rival their mother, to take on her role, to become, like her, the powerful sexual adult woman. The desire to 'be like mother', to learn through identifying with, or emulating parents or peers, is a normal aspect of development.

Although Klein herself concentrated exclusively on envy as an intra-psychic phenomenon, and barely mentioned family dynamics, some of her later collaborators theorised about possible environmental causes of excessive envy. Hanna Segal, in one of her studies of Klein, gives the example of the 'excessively narcissistic mother unable to cope with the infant's projections, and keeping herself as an idealised object' who then puts the infant into a constantly devalued position in relation to herself, thus increasing the child's envy of her.[17] Other writers (Salant-Schwartz,[18] Leslie Farber[19]) describe the way that envious parents may give the child the message, 'You have something special, but I hate you for it.' The child may then identify with the feeling of being very special, but repress the sense of being hated and envied. She may fantasise about being powerful and superior, while constantly engaging in a narcissistic search for admiration and respect from others. Parents who lack a strong sense of their own self-identity and value may become unduly sensitive to the child's feelings and reactions towards them. They may be unable to suspend their own need for admiration from others in order to respond to the child's need to have her emerging personality 'mirrored', to buid up an internalised sense of herself through seeing herself reflected in her parents' eyes. Instead, these envious, narcissistically vulnerable parents want the child to reflect them. Their insecurity and envy of their children – who, they feel, may have more fulfilling lives or create the sense of identity that they themselves lack – cause them constantly to undermine their children, spoiling their efforts and criticising destructively. Women's low social status within patriarchal culture inevitably affects our sense of identity and self-value; it may lead us to attempt to rely on our children for the recognition we do not get from elsewhere.

If the child is to value herself, to learn, be creative and make stable intimate relationships, she needs to have internalised consistent experiences in earliest infancy of feeling loved, satisfied, and reliably cared for. Intense deprivation, pain or frustration disrupt this process, and may cause the infant to develop strong doubts about her own goodness and worth, a deep-rooted sense of personal inadequacy which will cause her constantly to compare herself unfavourably with others. She may then, as Alice Miller describes, turn away from humiliation, pain or lack of understanding, hide her wishes and emotions behind a conforming 'false self' and envy others who do not have to 'walk on stilts' in a constant effort to win admiration, but are free to be 'average'.[20]

Melanie Klein stresses the role of primary envy rather than deprivation in preventing the development of a sense of self as lovable and valuable. In her view, the infant who is excessively envious and aggressive by nature, if not helped to tolerate these feelings and develop a stronger sense of herself as lovable and valuable, will come to feel that she has inside her something damaged, shredded, and poisonous. The source of goodness, the 'feeding breast' which she has come to experience as 'mean and grudging' has been spoiled by the aggressive and envious attacks she has made on it in her fantasies, and could no longer be experienced or internalised as an entirely 'good object'. She feels empty and hopeless, full of rubbish, beset by a sense of internal persecution and a fear of retaliation.

Although I think there are always environmental causes of envy, Klein's account indicates the powerful effects of the child's own painful, angry and envious reactions to frustration and humiliation on her developing sense of self. In one woman's nightmare, this unconscious persecutory aspect of herself was represented by a sweet young girl transformed by envy into a rotting, grimacing witch, with ragged clothes, stringy hair and a foul, poisonous smell, who lurked, snarling, behind a partition, waiting to attack.

The combination of early deprivation, hostility and envy may impair the child's ability to accept her own anger and aggression, to tolerate feeling both love and hatred towards the same person, and to establish a realistic image of the outside world. It becomes harder to assimilate satisfying experiences, to give, to receive with gratitude, to trust and co-operate.

The envious person cannot form truly equal relationships, since she is continually experiencing herself as inferior or superior to others. She either idealises other people or feels contempt for them. She has no sense of harmony inside herself, no concept of how an equal partnership would work, so she can find no middle ground in her external relationships. She can learn neither from others nor from her own experience, and so cannot develop her own internal world. The experience of being really dependent or of knowing less than others resonates with such an intolerable sense of inferiority, weakness and humiliation that the envious person can allow no one to be close to her, to help or teach her. She fears that she may be abandoned, or lose herself. She has extreme difficulty in absorbing knowledge, acquiring skills or opening herself up to new understandings. As Stephen Robinson points out, neither people nor objects can be 'used' imaginatively to nourish the envious person, who over-identifies with her own creations and cannot maintain a critical distance from the productions of others.[21] A vicious circle is then set up whereby the envious person's internal sense of worthlessness, deprivation and impoverishment is exacerbated by each actual experience of failure, so making external progress even more difficult and increasing her envy at the success and creativity of others.

However, if the child is cared for well enough to satisfy her own particular needs and suffers no serious physical or emotional setbacks, she will feel increasingly loving and grateful towards those who care for her, and her envy, competition and rivalry may actually be used as a spur to development. She will begin to understand that, through watching and emulating other children and adults, absorbing new experiences and learning from them, she can become more skilful, less helpless and dependent, and more like those she admires.

Psychoanalytic theories about analytic work with envy reflect the polarisation of views about its nature and origins. Klein sees envy as a fundamental cause of developmental difficulties. She describes the client's struggle to recognise and integrate envious destructiveness with infantile dependency, within the transference relationship with the therapist, as the most difficult and important part of any analysis. In contrast, Joffe sees envy as merely a visible sign of already existing and perhaps less accessible developmental disturbances. The envy is a symptom and a result of earlier difficulties, rather than a cause of them. Joffe describes these more fundamental anxieties and disturbances as the central focus of the therapy, rather than the envy itself, which may disappear of its own accord, he believes, once the underlying difficulties have been resolved. So, for instance, once the gifted person's internal conflicts and anxieties about creativity are understood and resolved, her envy of other people may diminish, since she may now be able to achieve more in her own life.

Although, in my view, envy is a result rather than a root cause of developmental disturbances, in practice it is difficult to distinguish cause and effect since once envy exists it exacerbates and creates problems. So, the client who continually sabotages therapeutic help may feel deeply envious, angry and guilty about her own feelings of destructiveness. It may be that her childhood experiences have, as in Jenny's case, left her feeling deeply lacking in personal confidence and unable to trust others. Her lack of internal security results in her being unable to risk external change, and this is exacerbated by envy, guilt and the repeated experience of failure.

Some people are obviously more envious than others. Nevertheless, every client in ongoing therapy will experience some degree of envy towards the therapist on whom she now depends for her future sense of psychological well-being, just as she once depended on her mother for her physical survival. The client's struggle to accept that she feels intense need and admiration, yet also hatred, envy and rivalry towards the therapist within the transference relationship may well, as Klein suggests, be the most painful but also the most potentially helpful part of the therapy.

In Kleinian theory, envy is associated with the earliest developmental phase, when the infant cannot yet integrate 'part-objects' – the terrifying breast, the hungry mouth, the reassuring lap – with the whole parent, and is not yet able to tolerate feelings of love and hate towards the same person. If, through the transference relationship, the client can come to accept and piece together all her different experiences of the therapist (as depriving yet also generous, as damaged by her attacks yet not destroyed) she may then be able to feel, as well as remorse, the desire to 'make up for' her aggression and gratitude for what she has received. In time, the therapist will come to be seen more clearly as she really is, a whole person in her own right. The client will then be able to experience herself as a more integrated person, no longer feeling so internally fragmented or divided. If the therapist, unlike the original parent, allows rage and anger without retaliating, the client, who can see that her feelings and fantasies cause no apparent damage, comes to feel, in Winnicott's terms, 'I can destroy the object and it will still survive.' She knows then that she also can survive the expression of her own envy and aggression, and she feels that now she can 'use' the therapist in order to develop a sense of herself as a separate and autonomous person.

Joffe emphasises that the existence of envy can, unlike depression, be seen as a sign of hope, since the envious person still entertains fantasies about having what she desires, and is not resigned to the discrepancy between what she is and what she wants to be. He stresses the importance for the therapist of pointing out not only the feelings of personal lack and hostility but also the admiration implicit in envy, since, if the idealised attributes are preserved from destruction, they can provide a basis for identification and the envied person can then be used as a model.[22] In this way, envy can lead to the development of a stronger sense of self, more satisfying relationships, and further achievements.

While these theoretical writings about envy are extremely relevant to the difficulties of the women I described earlier, the particular relevance of their own and their mothers' experience as women remains unexplored. Most theorists do acknowledge that envy has environmental causes and that what is envied varies between different groups and cultures, but we need to develop this by looking at the particular implications for women of psychoanalytic ideas about envy. Many links can be drawn between the envious and competitive feelings of the women described earlier in this chapter and the typical characteristics of women's psychological development within our society.

The experience of envy in therapy

If the destructive effects of envy are to play a less overwhelming role in our lives, we may have to examine deeply buried conflicts about ourselves, our relationships with others, about the possibility of failure or fulfilment. In my work with women I have learned that serious difficulties can arise if I don't help the apparently highly motivated, compliant, idealising client, such as Pauline, to recognise right from the beginning of therapy any underlying envy, scorn, humiliation and powerlessness she may feel in relation to myself and other people. It is equally important, however, not to lose sight of the fact that envy is always connected with admiration, dependency or love. Jenny and Pauline, whose histories I described earlier, came, as their therapy progressed, consciously to acknowledge and accept their feelings of envy and rivalry and to act on these feelings in ways that were constructive rather than destructive for themselves and, often, for other people too.

Pauline

Although Pauline had managed to create the kind of life she had wanted for herself, a part of her habitually spoiled any pleasure or satisfaction she might have derived from it. Since she could not assert her own needs at work or within the family, she turned her anger inwards, feeling miserable and depressed and envious of anyone who seemed to be happier or more sure of themselves. It was so difficult for her to express her long-pent-up envy, rage, powerlessness and humiliation that when this began to emerge, initially in quite dramatic outbursts, she would then miss sessions, so avoiding any possibility that I might retaliate destructively or that her aggression might destroy me. Whereas she had previously felt overwhelmingly trapped by a begrudging, controlling therapist—mother, she began to see me as slightly more helpful and less destructive of her moves towards independence. She began to feel more aware that she was a separate person with her own life to lead, rather than an extension of myself or her mother. She then felt more free to let me know the ways in which she still needed my help, rather than experiencing me in the same way as she had her mother, as someone who couldn't cope without having her near to control and dominate. This phase of her therapy was extremely disjointed, punctuated by long breaks and announcements that she was leaving immediately. But, as she was gradually able to see that I could tolerate both her aggression and her desire for independence, she became able to arrange her life in a way that would allow her more pleasure and intimacy. She also became more able to recognise her particular difficulties in standing up to and disagreeing with the important female figures in her own life.

Jenny

Jenny needed, in her therapy, to come to terms with two major fears—that her envy and aggression would damage me, or anyone else she became close to, and that if she allowed herself a fulfilling adult life, she would arouse my envy and lose my support and that of her family and friends. She watched me continuously for signs of physical or emotional deterioration, scrutinising me particularly closely after each holiday. Only when she had assured herself of my resilience against attack over a long period of time, could she allow herself to relax in my presence and use the therapy sessions to help herself. She gradually became more able to tolerate and contain her own feelings, with less of a need to re-create her own strong emotions in me and other people. Her overwhelming misery and frustration could then be channelled into attempts to change her own situation. She became less preoccupied with envious fantasies about me, and more able to create an image of the way she would like her own life to be. She began to express guilt and remorse towards both her mother and myself, feeling that she'd 'wasted' opportunities to develop, both in everyday life and in therapy. Around this time she realised that she could use aspects of her mother's life, and qualities she admired in me, as models to learn from. Changing and 'really using her life' would, she felt, be a form of reparation, a way of making up for the trials she'd caused. In fact, she was beginning to experience me, and therefore herself, in a slightly more integrated, less contradictory way.

Jenny had been so completely immobilised emotionally through fears of her own destructiveness that, although the recognition of these feelings was a long and tortuous process, the verbal expression of her envy and rage brought hope and relief. But, while misery and deprivation were familiar to her, success and independence were fraught with dangers. She hardly dared to tell me about her steps forward, lest I destroy them with criticism, or she took fright and sabotaged them. Now that she was more independent, she feared that I would become ill, as her mother had done when she had first talked of leaving home, or that she would arouse my envy and retaliation. But gradually Jenny stopped presenting herself as so pathetic, and increasingly developed her own interests. However, she now feared that since she was no longer so 'interestingly neurotic' she would become less attractive to men, and women would envy her increased emotional strength. But as she began to feel more internally secure and self-reliant, she also became more able to risk change and competition in order to get more of what she wanted in her life.

Although competition is sometimes described as undesirable, in fact our possibilities in life are severely restricted if we are totally unable or unwilling to compete or to put ourselves in a position where we may inspire feelings of envy or rivalry in others. The ability to compete (which is not the same as obsessive rivalry) is then a necessary and desirable attribute. For instance, in order to find almost any form of employment at present, it is often necessary to compete quite fiercely and any challenging or fulfilling activity, whether it be bringing up children, writing books, or climbing mountains, may well inspire envy or feelings of rivalry in others.

Jenny and Pauline's difficulties in experiencing themselves as worthwhile, strongly defined, independent people, able to stand up for themselves and if necessary to compete for what they wanted, can be related both to patterns of women's socialisation within our society, and to girls' experience within the mother–daughter relationship.

Women's work both inside and outside the home has traditionally been undervalued. Childcare, highly responsible work requiring great dedication, is carried out in isolation, with very little support, social recognition or validation. It is not surprising, then, that many mothers invest enormous emotional energy in their children, looking particularly to their daughters to reflect them, to provide the support, sympathy, love and respect of which they feel deprived elsewhere. This is part of the external social reality behind the preoccupation many women have with the fear of their mothers' envy. Just as they may have been making their first early teenage steps towards psychological separation while still needing their mothers' support and approval, many women seem to have become keenly aware of a feeling that their mothers envied and resented their youthful attractiveness and future opportunities. It is particularly difficult for a daughter to feel free psychologically to move towards adult womanhood if, like Jenny, she has experienced some emotional insecurity or deprivation in childhood and her mother is making it clear, consciously or unconsciously, that she doesn't look forward to a future without her daughter.

Women's fear of other women's envy may reflect both social reality, and the actual individual experience of having had an envious mother but, at a psychological level, it is also a way of avoiding both their own envious feelings and their unconscious conflicts about competition, success and failure. The woman who fears that she will provoke envy and lose friends if she becomes thinner and more sexually attractive may find that reality bears this out. On the other hand, this fear may be a projection of her own denied envy of thin women, and a way of avoiding unconscious conflicts about intimacy, dependency and sexuality.

Changing social and political attitudes and circumstances obviously affect women's experience. So Joan felt she grew up without role-models and now feels part of an 'in-between' generation, unsure whether to identify herself with her working-class mother, or her middle-class peers. Current contradictory pressures – increased unemployment, combined with changing assumptions about women's work outside the home, may create new feelings of inadequacy which can be expressed in heightened envy and rivalry between women.

The experience of being a second-class citizen within patriarchal culture is, as many feminists have pointed out, internalised psychologically as a 'sense of lack', of 'something missing', that is, a sense of self as whole, strong and valuable. Some version of this sense of incompleteness is, according to Janine Chasseguet-Smirgel,[23] found in infants of both sexes, and is the result of 'narcissistic wounds' created by the experience of overwhelming dependence on an all-powerful mother who is 'capable of everything and possesses every valuable attribute'. The infant develops an internal 'terrifying maternal imago', largely caused by its own resentment of these wounds, and an ever-generous, loving, protective imago, which will only be internalised if the infant has 'good enough' care and will then reflect more of the mother's real attributes. Unlike boys, girls cannot compensate for these narcissistic wounds and assert their autonomy from their mothers by demonstrating that they have something which is not only different, but also more highly valued in our society. Women's tendency to remain more in touch with early infantile experiences with their mothers and their difficulty in differentiating themselves psychologically are reflected in the painful struggles of Jenny and Pauline to separate themselves from the internalised images of their mothers through the transference relationship with me.

While men can further compensate for internalised infantile humiliations and losses through developing an image of themselves as capable, creative and successful in some area of life, it is not so easy for women to make up for their own feelings of lack in this way. Women's traditional area of creativity –

giving birth to and nurturing children is not only socially undervalued but (as Sheila Ernst points out) demands from women the capacity to remain in touch with those very areas of infantile experience from which the male role offers a possible form of escape. Nor is it so easy for women to develop a sense of their own value in the external world of work, since internal conflicts, such as those I describe in this chapter, may well reinforce and interact with real practical obstacles and discriminatory attitudes. Many of the women I have described were attempting to develop aspects of themselves regarded as traditionally male, as well as those considered female; to become whole, integrated women with personal authority in the outside world, as well as developing capacities to nurture and be close to others. In childhood, the girl's ability to develop and integrate these different aspects of herself will be influenced not only by her parents' conscious attitudes, but also by what they unconsciously communicate about the male and female parts of themselves. Similarly in therapy the woman will be influenced by her therapist's conscious and unconscious feelings and attitudes about the possibility of women achieving a sense of personal autonomy and developing and integrating 'male' as well as 'female' aspects of themselves.

The girl's early infantile experience of identification with her mother's receptivity, sensitivity and nurturing qualities may partly account for her ability to remain in touch with her own inner processes and those of others. Feelings and fantasies connected with envy and inadequacy may then be closer to a woman's conscious awareness, more integrated with everyday experience, than they are in men. While this means that she may not, as an adult, be able to cut off from and deny these feelings absolutely, and so may not appear to 'manage' as well as men do in the external world, the fact that she is much more in touch with this aspect of herself may help her to integrate and accept it, and so develop the more genuine strengths that come from building on her own internal resources.

For Pauline, Jenny and Joan, as for many other women, it was the aggressive aspects of envy and rivalry that were expressed most indirectly. While some women use aggression as a defence against vulnerability, many women completely deny and disown their anger and critical feelings, their contempt, rage and violence. This not only inhibits closeness, as shown in Pauline's therapy, but often makes it difficult for women to speak out for themselves or act on dissatisfactions assertively. Although many women can disagree with and even compete with men, amongst women there is often a shared terror of even the mildest disagreement. This seems to reflect internal fears of retaliation and persecution. A women's group may react with horror to a difference of opinion amongst members, rallying protectively around the woman who they feel has been 'attacked'. The ability to differ with open confidence requires a feeling of internal separateness and independence from each other that women often do not have.

For many women, the only way of getting in touch with their own needs, feelings and desires is by identifying with those of others. Jenny, when she projected her own fantasies and wishes into an idealised image of my lifestyle, provided a typical example of the way in which women attempt to arrive at a sense of who they are by comparing, contrasting and evaluating themselves in relation to other women and to internalised images of their own mother.

The account of Joan and Olivia's friendship illustrates the way in which women's relationships with each other may reflect patterns present in many mother–daughter relationships. There may be strong feelings of closeness, even a sense of fusion. Women readily identify with each other, especially around experiences of inadequacy and vulnerability but intense love and admiration may suddenly reverse into their counterparts – envy, hatred and rivalry. Eichenbaum and Orbach in *Understanding Women* describe the way that women hold on to the safety of their second-class status and use it as a connecting link with each other. They quote from Simone de Beauvoir who says in *The Second Sex*, 'Women are comrades in captivity for each other. They help one another endure their prison, even help one another prepare for escape.' But, as Eichenbaum and Orbach point out, one woman's escape can be experienced as another's betrayal, and women unconsciously collude in holding themselves and each other back from greater personal fulfilment. 'Deeply instilled in each woman is an unconscious knowledge of the thresholds she cannot cross without arousing the anger and envy of other women.' Focusing on this may be a way of avoiding unconscious anxieties about competing with and perhaps triumphing over their own mothers, as well as an expression of guilt and fear about breaking with deeply instilled feminine stereotypes. Used as they are to ranking each other on a scale of attributes which varies but always includes sexual attractiveness, now, ironically, many women admit to a terror of being judged not to be, look or sound 'feminist' enough. Eichenbaum and Orbach describe the way each woman may feel depression, self-hatred and hopelessness in relation to others, while at the same time longing to be in their shoes. 'Perhaps', they say, 'the most painful aspect of this cycle of insecurity and competition is that women experience these feelings individually and yet they are common to millions of women.'[24]

Apart from the immediate relief of acknowledging long-prohibited feelings and seeing that both we and other women can survive their expression, there are many long-term psychological, social and political benefits to be gained from understanding and accepting our own envy and rivalry. The envious person focuses on others, rather than on herself. Through re-owning our own envious fantasies we can become more sure about our own desires, can concentrate on our own sense of direction. When we begin to recognise the extent of our own envy, competitiveness and aggression, we gain access to a previously inaccessible aspect of ourselves, a source of potential strength. We can then use our aggression and rivalry in our own and perhaps in other people's interests, rather than sabotaging ourselves and others with our unacknowledged envy. If, as many women do, we rely entirely on expressions of vulnerability and misery in order to get our needs met, then, by facing up to our own aggression and our fear of arousing envy and hostility if we succeed in any way, our sense of ourselves will change radically.

Once we acknowledge our feelings of inferiority and our rivalry towards those who know more than we do or possess skills and capacities we lack, we will find ourselves more able to learn, to accept and use help gracefully. If we feel more sure of ourselves, needing less to compensate for feelings of inferiority with arrogant self-assertion, we will be able to form more genuinely equal relationships, based on openness and co-operation. We will become more creative, less afraid to compete, less concerned about the risks of failure, or the effects of success.

It is particularly important that envy and rivalry be recognised and expressed in both emotional and working relationships between women. The more we come to terms with our own envy and aggression the more capable we become of having genuinely loving relationships which can also be more productive, more stable and resilient. Women are particularly able to nurture and support each other's vulnerabilities, to be sensitive to each other's difficulties. But we may also, without consciously realising it, hold each other back from greater independence and fulfilment. We need to become more able to accept the ways in which we are different from other women, to realise that we have our own unique resources and disadvantages, and that in order to be honest about who we are and what we think, we may have to risk conflict. We need to become able to support each other in being strong and independent, while recognising that, although we may sometimes arouse envy by our success, we may also have to watch other women doing and attaining things that we can never have or do.

Some envious feelings have to be accepted, since they are caused by unchangeable personal or social inequalities. But once we are more aware of our own individual envy we can then understand more about the social and political implications of this emotion. Stephen Robinson sees our culture as 'envy-based', in its denial of need, feeling and dependency, and connects this with contemporary attacks on our social and physical environment through pollution, resource abuse, and ultimately the threat of nuclear war.[25] Within feminist theory there has been a constant preoccupation with this life-denying tendency in our culture, and women have been in the forefront of campaigns and political actions against these threats to ourselves and our environment. This does not mean, however, that women are essentially benign, that we have no responsibility for this destructiveness, no urge to damage, spoil or steal. It is important that we do not blind ourselves to our collusion in such social and political violence.

Envy attacks the capacitv to change. This capacity requires the strength and courage to open ourselves up and be intensely vulnerable, to learn from our experience. It is different from learning *about* things, from the external accretion of knowledge which, at its worst, can mean acquiring dead facts by rote. If we feel that our psychological structures are too flimsy, that we will either collapse or lose ourselves if we become open enough to learn, or to become really intimate with others, we will not only maintain a rigid psychological position, but also be unable to contribute towards any really creative political communication or change.

Acknowledgments

I'd like to thank all the people close to me who gave me practical and emotional support and discussed ideas with me during the long gestation of this chapter. I'd also like to thank Margot Waddell and Eleanor Armstrong-Perlman who read a later draft and gave me very detailed and valuable comments and criticisms. Finally, I'd like to express gratitude to my mother, who loves to listen.

Marie Maguire

Notes

1. The first quotation is from Janine Chasseguet-Smirgel, *Female Sexuality*, Maresfield, London, 1985, p.118; the second from a woman psychotherapy client.
2. In this chapter I assume that the child's first mothering relationship is with a woman. While I recognise that this may not always be the case, it has been the experience of all the women I have so far seen as psychotherapy clients.

3. Quoted by Melanie Klein in *Envy and Gratitude and Other Essays*, Delta edition., Dell Co., New York, 1977, p.189 (originally published 1957).

4. This reference I owe to Leslie Farber, *Lying, Despair, Jealousy, Envy, Sex, Drugs and the Good Life*, Basic Books, New York, 1976, from his essay, 'faces of envy'.

5. Klein, *Envy and Gratitude and Other Essays*, p.189.

6. H. Schoeck, *Envy: a theory of social behaviour*, Harcourt, Brace, New York, 1966.

7. Details of the clinical material I have drawn on in this chapter have been altered in the interests of confidentiality.

8. Klein, op. cit., p.218.

9. Chasseguet-Smirgel, *Female Sexuality*, p.118.

10. Klein, op. cit., pp. 216-20. In these pages Klein gives a detailed account of ways in which people defend themselves against envy.

11. Sigmund Freud, *New Introductory Lectures on Psycho-analysis*, Pelican, Harmondsworth, 1973, p.155.

12. W.G. Joffe, 'A critical review of the status of the envy concept', *International Journal of Psycho-Analysis*, 50, 1969, p.533.

13. Klein, op. cit., .

14. D.W. Winnicott, 'Creativity and its origins' in *Playing and Reality*, Pelican, Harmondsworth, 1971, p.96.

15. Luise Eichenbaum and Susie Orbach, *Understanding Women*, Penguin, Harmondsworth, 1985.

16. Klein, op. cit., p.183.

17. Hanna Segal, *Klein*, Fontana, London, 1979, p.147.

18. N. Salant-Schwartz, *Narcissism and Character Transformation*, Inner City Books, New York, 1982.

19. Leslie Farber, 'The faces of envy', in *Lying, Despair, Jealousy, Sex, Drugs and the Good Life*.

20. Alice Miller, *The Drama of the Gifted Child and the Search for the True Self*, Faber & Faber, London, 1983, p.59.

21. Stephen Robinson, 'The parent to the child', in B. Richards (ed.), *Capitalism and Infancy*, Free Association Books, London, 1984.

22. Joffe, 'A critical review of the status of the envy concept'.

23. Chasseguet-Smirgel, *Female Sexuality*.

24. Eichenbaum and Orbach, *Understanding Women*, pp.142-4.

25. Robinson, 'The parent to the child'.

6
Abortion – a woman's right to feel

Abortion is experienced by women in many different ways. Post-abortion groups at the WTC were set up to give women a chance to explore their feelings about having had an abortion in a group setting with other women who had also had an abortion.

The aim of this chapter is to draw up a theoretical analysis based on my working experience with women in these post-abortion groups. This will include an attempt at understanding the external political situation and our own social conditioning as women in a patriarchal society, as well as the internal expression of it in women's individual experience with pregnancy and abortion.

Before beginning, I would like to clarify the three different levels I will be talking about. The first and most immediate level is the experience itself, what actually happens, and the feelings surrounding it. The second level is that of the unconscious. These two levels obviously interact and overlap in everything we do, even if we are unaware of it in our everyday behaviour. Many people live their lives without having to recognise the existence of the unconscious. It may take an unpleasant or painful experience such as an unwanted pregnancy and its termination to force a person to face the fact that there may be other forces at work besides the apparently straightforward and obvious ones. These two worlds have their own languages: the language of common sense, which we use to discuss events, feelings, issues, relationships, etc., in a day-to-day factual way; and the language of the unconscious which involves unconscious motives and meanings as well as patterns that we carry with us from our childhood.

The third level is the social level. Neither families nor individuals exist in isolation, but are influenced by the society in which they function, by its norms, morals and value systems. It is impossible to understand personal behaviour, both conscious and unconscious, without linking it to women's conditioning and position in our society. The experience of abortion is one in which these three realities meet – conscious, unconscious, and social; this chapter attempts to show the connections between them.

I would also like to acknowledge two points which have affected my understanding of abortion. Firstly, my own experience of abortion was very painful. This may at times in my work have biased me towards looking at the painful aspects of having an abortion. Secondly, the women I have worked with, both individually and in groups, sought help because they also had had difficult and painful experiences.

What I have to say will not necessarily apply to all women. And my analysis only represents one aspect of a large spectrum of issues, both personal and political, most of which are very controversial in a changing society. Some issues I can only acknowledge and not discuss in detail. They include, for example, the unsatisfactory nature of available contraceptive methods, and the lack of choice for many women about whether to have a baby, because of their lack of social, economic, practical or personal support.

Before the 1967 Abortion Act thousands of women took the legal and medical risks of backstreet abortions resulting in many cases in severe physical complications. Much of the effort and energy of the women's movement went into fighting an impossible situation.[1] Abortion was against the law, a taboo, and had to be kept a secret. The 1967 Abortion Act was an enormous step forward in the political battle – it has, at least, given grounds for many abortions to be performed legally. Yet liberal as it may have seemed, it in no way challenged the medical and moral hierarchy upon which many of society's attitudes to abortion are based. The law may be open to a liberal interpretation in both the public and the individual's eye, but it only allows abortion if there are sufficient medical or social grounds and this has to be judged by doctors. It does not allow for abortion on demand. Some doctors interpret it in this sense but others hold it to mean that only women in dire emotional and social circumstances should be given abortions. Women are 'free' to have abortions, but the power is left firmly in the hands of the medical hierarchy. This has led to huge anomalies, allowing individual doctors to decide according to their own individual bias, be it in relation to religion, race, class, physical appearance or marital status. Taken to its extreme, this can mean that a working-class woman may be discriminated against whereas a well-educated woman may have a better chance of convincing her doctor to allow her an abortion.

In 1975 a first attempt was made at restricting the law and it was at this point that the National Abortion Campaign was formed. It was set up not just to fight proposed restrictions but also to assert positively 'a woman's right to choose'. At that time it was still too 'dangerous' to talk about the painful emotions surrounding abortion because the anti-abortion pressure groups had monopolised the emotional and moral ground. It was they who spelt out the emotionally painful aspects of having an abortion, they who argued that abortion was killing. Because of these threats to women's right to abortion, it was almost impossible for feminists to engage with the emotionally difficult aspects of abortion or the complex moral issues involved. And it was hard to realise that acknowledging the painful and damaging aspects of abortion does not invalidate women's needs for freely available and safe abortion. (This is interesting in terms of the cultural denial of pain – the way in which early feminism could not really take on board both women's past pain and the pain which making changes might entail.)

Since 1975 restrictive bills have been a regular occurrence. As the years have gone by, however, the threat – while not disappearing – has lessened. This has allowed women involved in the abortion campaign to begin to look at the situation more broadly. Women have started to say that the slogans no longer correspond to their experience and to the very wide range of issues raised by a campaign for full reproductive rights: the issues, for example, of black women being encouraged to have abortions, or to be sterilised as a condition of having an abortion; of infertility; or of lesbians and artificial insemination.

The campaign has therefore had to widen its interest to other aspects of reproductive rights, and in 1983 the Women's Reproductive Rights Campaign was formed. The legal and political pressure having slightly declined, women were able to turn their attention to their own feelings, to explore the effects of these past years as well as the emotional aspects of having an abortion. There are now more and more post-abortion groups in which women can break the secrecy that has been imposed upon them for years and look at their feelings before, during and after abortion. There has also been a new recognition on the part of the pregnancy advisory agencies of the need for counselling not only *before* but also *after* an abortion.

Some feminist writers have pinpointed the complex and difficult situation women find themselves in:

> Abortion is hardly the 'final triumph' envisaged by all, or the final stage of the revolution. There are deep questions beneath and beyond this, such as why should women be in the situation of unwanted pregnancy at all? Some women see abortion as a humiliating procedure . . . few if any feminists are deceived in this matter although male proponents of the repeal of abortion laws tend often to be short sighted in this respect, confusing the feminist revolution with the sexual revolution. . . . [2]

And again: 'The demand for legalized abortion, like the demand for contraception, has been represented as a form of irresponsibility, a refusal by women to confront their moral destiny, a trivialization or evasion of great issues of life and death. The human facts, however, are hardly frivolous.' [3] Here Adrienne Rich gives examples of the risks women go through in attempting to terminate their own pregnancy when denied a legal abortion. 'To become pregnant with an unwanted child', Adrienne Rich says,

> is no light experience. Guilt about abortion can serve as the channel for other, older feelings of guilt, and the need to atone. It can also be the result of a life-long exposure to the

idea that abortion is murder. If a woman feels her guilt or depression as a kind of punishment, she may try to disavow such feelings. It is crucial however, in abortion, as in every other experience, that women take seriously the enterprise of finding out what we do feel instead of what we have been told we must feel.[4]

It is important therefore that both painful, 'negative' feelings as well as 'positive' feelings should be discussed. It is these feelings, expressed by women with whom I have worked, that I would like to present throughout this chapter.

The myth of motherhood

One of the most important and oppressive aspects of our social reality is the myth of motherhood which becomes, through conditioning – in the broader sense of discovering one's own gender – a part of the inner world of every woman. This myth and its reflection in a woman's inner world is part of the reason why the experience of abortion is so painful for women.

Many of the myths in our Judaeo–Christian society are to do with the bond between mother and baby. Take, for example, the story of Solomon. Two mothers both claimed ownership of the same baby. When Solomon judged that the baby should be cut in two, one woman agreed but the real mother said 'No – she can have him, let him not die.' Both motherhood and unconditional love between mother and baby are hereby glorified: the true mother can only be recognised by her unconditional love.

The 'myth of motherhood', the portrayal of women as essentially mothers, takes place on several levels. On a social level, in a society in which the nuclear family is an idealised and desired unit, women's role is primarily as mother. Furthermore, in terms of their relationship with people around them, women are brought up to become mothers, the carers of others, meeting other people's needs, often having to put their own needs in second place. Mothers thus produce daughters who will repeat this pattern. Lastly, in terms of her deepest sense of herself as an individual, a woman's identity is traditionally invested in becoming a wife and mother and that is where she is to find her sense of self. Added to this is a woman's biological potential as a mother and the unconscious processes that are formulated with the interaction of all these factors. The picture that emerges to a woman of herself is that motherhood equals womanhood.

This is further complicated by the fact that psychoanalytic theories have increased the idealisation of women's maternal role by emphasising the crucial importance of the mother–child relationship to the child's psychological development and internal world. This creates still another idealised standard that women can seldom if ever achieve. Winnicott's term of the 'good enough mother' comes as a great relief. In reality, being a wife and a mother is far from an ideal situation. In the role of mother women are devalued as people in their own right, frustrated and unappreciated.

In an attempt to change women's situation in our society and to address the kind of frustrations they experience, the women's movement has helped to create alternatives for women. Women are making different choices in their lives: to be single, not to have children, to have children in different situations, such as lesbian couples, single mothers and so on. Feminism has overall brought about a change in women's awareness of their sense of self, their identity as women and their creativity in the world.

However, the more traditional picture is still very powerful for many women – understandably, given the fact that these social and psychological myths have been operating for so long and are underpinned by the power relations of our society. Many women still see motherhood as the most creative act in their lives, still equate womanhood with motherhood and still invest their sense of self and identity in that role alone. Far from wanting to reduce the importance and very creative nature of having children, I wish to emphasise that it is not the *only* way in which women can express their creative powers.

Moreover, for all of us there is no simple answer to such questions as: What does it mean to be a woman? Who is feminine? What is femininity? How and when does a woman become a 'real woman'? Given this lack of a clear concept of femininity, it is not surprising that motherhood – that tangibly creative, practical role – is grasped at as a prime symbol of femininity.

It thus becomes clearer why abortion is such a painful and difficult experience for so many women. If motherhood means womanhood, what does abortion which is its opposite, its 'negation' mean in terms of external – social and internal – personal definitions? It cannot fail to raise many issues about femininity and womanhood, for the woman concerned as well as for society at large.

I will talk later in this chapter about the emotions that emerge as a result of this conditioning in women who have had abortions. Here I just want to pose some of the basic conflicts involved in that experience. Women have expressed this in sentences like 'I feel I am not a woman. I feel I have lost the chance to become one.' (Considering the exaggerated danger of infertility claimed by the medical profession, this can seem a real fear.) Or 'I did not fulfil my creativity, myself.' For many women the issue is therefore not motherhood *per se*, but motherhood as a symbol of their fertility and thus of their womanhood. I realise that this is more true for women who have not yet had children, but I have also worked with mothers who still carried these feelings, as if they had spoilt their womanhood or had doubts about whether they ever had or deserved it in the first place.

As we have seen, an important part of the myth of motherhood is the picture of an unconditional, all-giving, all-good, never-harming mother, and of an eternal, incomparable, inseparable bond between mother and child. The mother will sacrifice her life and happiness to save that of her child. She will always love it and will never do anything to harm it. Without ignoring the very powerful, intense and unique relationship that does exist and develop between mother and child, the myth sets up an extremely beautiful image which allows no ambivalence. No murderous, angry, hateful, negative emotions, least of all no 'killing'. Many of the women I have worked with have expressed feelings that they have 'killed' their baby and experienced deep feelings of guilt and sadness to the point of relating to the abortion as 'murder'. Eileen Fairweather, in her article 'The feelings behind the slogans'[5] puts the argument about the issue of killing in a very clear way: 'One of the defensive slogans the National Abortion Campaign used is that the foetus is a potential human life incapable of independent existence'. Another slogan was, 'The egg is not a chicken, an acorn is not a tree, a foetus is not a baby . . . ' 'Why', she asks,

> do we have to make support for women's right to choose dependent on seeing the foetus as no more than a bunch of splitting cells? In doing so, we lose potential supporters and that includes those women who have had an abortion, but think of it as a killing. Some women experience nothing but relief after an abortion. Others only feel guilty because they don't feel guilty. But for many women it is not so simple . . .
>
> The 'potential human life' argument implies that a woman is merely suffering from feminine fancy and sexist conditioning if she feels she has in any way 'killed' her foetus/baby. It may have seemed the most 'revolutionary' position, but it was not always helpful to women, since it denies so many of women's actual experiences and feelings.

Therefore there are many different ways of viewing abortion – as killing, as a simple removal of tissue or as the termination of a potential but not actual life. Whatever one's views, the important thing is to acknowledge these views and for each woman to be allowed to express her own.

For many women, the reality is that a potential life has been terminated. This reality, however, will echo in each woman's feelings and internal experience in a different way. The knowledge will have a different mark on her psychic life and fantasy world, according to her life experiences, her beliefs, current circumstances and emotional make-up. It is peculiar, then, that women as a group and as individuals are stigmatised, accused of murder and made to feel guilty about it, when at the same time socialised mass murder such as men going to

war or shooting at people in demonstrations is socially acceptable and permitted, or at least is not defined as murder, with
blame attaching to individuals.

Abortion as an expression of internal conflict

Here I would like to discuss how women's unconscious life is
reflected in the experience of pregnancy and abortion. In this
part of the chapter I therefore talk mainly in terms of the
unconscious. So that when talking about the element of
'choice' in getting pregnant and having an abortion it is not a
'conscious' choice that I am referring to.

Pregnancy and abortion may be a 'straightforward' situation – but they may also be the product of all sorts of unconscious conflicts. The important point is to try to understand
the unconscious motivation so that we are better able to act
freely in our lives, causing less pain to ourselves through being
compelled to act out these conflicts without awareness of what
they are or how to deal with them in a direct way.

There are some women, of course, who do not use contraception or use it incorrectly, who really do want a baby but
may not consciously admit it. On becoming pregnant they go
through with it and have the baby. This means that there is a
difference between women who just 'want' to be pregnant,
and those who actually want to have a baby.

I believe that for some women, getting pregnant and having
an abortion is one *joint* experience. Let me try to make this
point clearer. If such a woman were asked what she would do
in the event of becoming pregnant, she would know more or
less what she would intend to do. In the light of this knowledge, not using contraception is taking a risk if she knows her
circumstances do not allow her to have a baby at that time.
The risk includes both getting pregnant and having an abortion. Here I am mainly talking about women who do not use
contraception or use it incorrectly, not about contraceptive
failure.

Let us take, for example, a student in the middle of her final year at university. Her exams are due soon. She lives in a squat and can hardly manage on her grant. Her relationship with her boyfriend is very rocky; they have split up recently and are assessing their relationship. They spend the evening together and unexpectedly go back to his place, she having left her cap at home, and he saying, 'Oh, it will be OK.' She is somewhat drunk and excited and forgets about contraception.

Another example is a woman who has just had a baby and is intending to go back to work which is, for her, of prime importance. She is using the low-dose pill, knowing it has to be taken at the same time every day. She forgets to take the pill one day, has intercourse and the next day remembers and takes two pills on the same day. Obviously it takes two to have 'unsafe' sex, but it is the woman who usually carries the consequence.

All such examples have an unconscious meaning. Though the word unconscious is widely used in day-to-day speech, it is important to emphasise that it really means a person is completely unaware of their unconscious feelings, conflicts, meanings. The assumption I am making here is that many women who do not use contraception or who use it incorrectly do so for unconscious psychological reasons which include becoming pregnant and terminating the pregnancy. If you like, there is an element of 'choice', i.e., a woman unconsciously 'chooses' to become pregnant.

I would like to state here that this concept of 'choice' in a woman becoming pregnant could easily be used to blame women and abuse them in a way I strongly object to. My aim in introducing it is not to blame. On the contrary, I believe that through understanding the conflicts underlying her actions a woman can deal with these in a more direct way and be able to take responsibility for what she felt and what has happened. Through this she can gain more control over her life and understand consciously the choices that she faces, thus not having to act out these conflicts in such a painful way as having an abortion or several abortions. In psychological terms, the more the unconscious can be made conscious, the more the woman is in control of her life.

A woman's body

Before we look at the different meanings of these conflicts it is important to make clear how much a woman's body becomes a vehicle for the indirect expression of them. There are many examples of this, but getting pregnant and having an abortion is a very painful way.

Throughout patriarchal mythology, dream symbolism, theology, language, two ideas flow side by side: one, that the female body is impure, corrupt, the site of discharges, bleeding dangerous to masculinity, a source of moral and physical contamination, 'The devil's gateway'. On the other hand, as a mother the woman is beneficial, sacred, pure, asexual, nourishing, and the physical potential for mother-hood. This same body with its bleeding and its mysteries is her single destiny and justification in life. These two ideas have been deeply internalized in women, even in the most independent of us, those of us who seem to lead the freest of lives. In order to maintain two such notions, each in its con-tradictory purity, the masculine imagination has had to divide, to see us, and force us to see ourselves as polarized into good and evil, fertile or barren, pure or impure and all these fantasies are symbolized in and centred around a woman's body.

This is only one of the social contradictions that women have internalized as 'facts of life' and internally, in silence and solitude have been made to carry the pain of those inter-nalized notions and the burden of social guilt as their own.[6]

The way in which social conditioning affects women's percep-tion of their bodies is again illustrated in *Outside In . . . Inside Out* by Susie Orbach and Luise Eichenbaum.

Women's social position means that the woman's sphere of influence is limited and that it is confined very much within her own home – if you like within her own body. A woman's body is her primary asset in the world, for with it she gains a man, a family, a home, a place in the world. A woman's body therefore, is integral to her social position of wife and mother. At the same time, as we know, certain aspects of a woman's life inevitably cause conflict which it may be impossible to express. The distress a woman feels, the conflicts she experiences, the taboos against her longings often show themselves not surprisingly in woman's terrain: her body. A woman may unconsciously express her distress through her body.[7]

Getting pregnant and having an abortion is one such expression of distress.

Society and life in general are full of contradictions and conflicts for both women and men but as Jean Baker Miller suggests: 'Conflict has been a taboo area for women and for key reasons. Women are supposed to be the quintessential accommodators, mediators, the adapters and soothers. All of us, but women especially, are taught to see conflict as something frightening and evil.'[8] Women are not expected, allowed or even given 'normative channels' to express conflicts. So, women will more often than not find indirect ways to deal with this conflict.

Ambivalence

The unconscious working out of ambivalent feelings about ourselves can be deeply involved in the experience of abortion.

Ambivalent feelings, similar to conflicts, are often expressed and dealt with in indirect ways. Ambivalence seems to be unbearable and not fully incorporated into our lives. We often strive for perfection, and see things in terms of good or bad, right or wrong, all extreme attitudes that leave little space for ambivalence or for an understanding or tolerance of both sides. This attitude provides neither the permission to have ambivalent feelings, nor the ability to tolerate the anxiety they produce. Because of a woman's emotional state when pregnant and the very rich fantasy she experiences in that state, many characteristics of her own internal world are projected into the new entity that is now growing inside her. Sometimes, the foetus will have projected on to it bad aspects of the woman, for example ugliness, nastiness, stupidity. This means that if an abortion is done, a 'bad' part of the woman is got rid of and she may experience relief. This relief can, however, only be temporary. As human beings we are all bound to have feelings of 'badness' inside us which make us uncomfortable. One way of avoiding dealing with these feelings ourselves is to project them on to others, as in common racist attitudes, but these feelings do not go away. Through projecting the feelings of 'badness' on to the foetus and then having the abortion, a woman may unconsciously fantasise that she has rid herself of those feelings. Unfortunately the feelings will return in full force as it is not possible to rid oneself of them in that way. If, however, what is projected on to the foetus are her 'good', tender, warm, loving feelings, to have to separate from these because of an abortion will also be extremely painful and cause great distress. What actually needs to happen is an acknowledgment that both 'bad' and 'good' feelings belong to the self.

The acknowledgment of ambivalent feelings toward the pregnancy is thus very important as well as difficult when the pregnancy and the woman's relation to it are on a fantasy level.

Relationship with mother

The relationship with the mother is a most important element affecting both getting pregnant in the first place, and the decision as to whether or not to terminate.

In *Inside Out . . . Outside In* Susie Orbach and Luise Eichenbaum spell out very clearly the well-known way in which babies are born in the parents' (especially the mother's) expectation that they will be a source of unconditional love. I have extracted a few points relevant to my discussion. Women learn to transform the need to care for themselves into caring for others. Inside every woman there is a repressed, arrested, dependent part, a figure whose needs were never sufficiently attended to, recognised or cared for. This part of her is forever hungry for that recognition, care and acceptance that she never got enough of from her mother. The woman is ashamed of this part, believing it to be bad, unacceptable, weak, and not to be expressed or even considered. This may create a conflict. The conflict is magnified and comes to the fore when, say, in an intimate relationship with a partner the opportunity opens up for that deprived childhood figure to be seen, recognised and cared for. This opportunity is both attractive and terrifying for the woman considering how unacceptable she feels it to be and how repressed it has been.

One indirect way of dealing with these conflicts and fears is by externalising this needy, uncared-for childhood figure and transforming it to a fantasy of a figure who will provide unconditional love, bond, care, for example – a baby. The woman may act on this fantasy by getting pregnant. In other words, wanting to be cared for is translated into wanting to care for. (In her chapter on separation Sheila Ernst describes this whole issue of merging with and separation from the mother.) The prospect, however, of being the actual carer of a real baby can be so overwhelming that the woman decides to have an abortion.

What other aspects of the mother–daughter relationship might affect a woman's decision of whether or not to have an abortion? Dionora Pines, in an article on the effects of early psychic life on pregnancy and abortion, analyses the relationship with the mother and how it affects a woman in pregnancy and abortion.[9] (In the article she talks about a first pregnancy.) The first point she makes is, as I have often found in my work, that there is a marked distinction between the wish to become pregnant, and the wish to bring a live child into the world and become a mother. What seems to dictate the difference for each individual woman is her own early experience with her mother. When a woman is pregnant, she often finds herself going back to the feelings and fantasies of early infancy, like being a baby in her mother's womb. In experiencing this regression, she identifies with her mother's feelings towards her as a baby and with her own feelings as herself in the womb, or as a tiny infant in an almost symbiotic fusion with her mother.

The particular feelings that she had as an infant will influence her feelings towards the foetus and whether or not she wishes to carry on with the pregnancy. For example, if she feels that her mother was blissful and loving towards her as a baby then she is likely to have similar feelings towards her own baby. If, however, her mother was deeply ambivalent about having a baby, her attitude towards her own baby may include ambivalence, insecurity, conflict, and in interaction with other aspects of her life (her partner, the support she gets and her external reality) may determine her decision for or against an abortion. For some women pregnancy may be one of the most enriching times of their lives. For others, it is a painful and frightening experience.

Dionora Pines then goes on to explain how separation from the mother and becoming an individual, separate person is a life-long process for women. Pregnancy is an important point in this process.

If the woman is re-experiencing her own intra-uterine life and her own birth, many feelings and fantasies from that period will be revived. She will feel anxious, vulnerable, angry, overwhelmed with love, for no apparent reason. Positive and negative feelings and aspects of the self will therefore be projected on to the unseen foetus as if it were an extension of her self. Pregnancy provides many women with an alternative to resolving these conflicts directly. These conflicts may affect whether the foetus will be given life or physically rejected through abortion.

Lastly, a woman who feels unseparated from her mother will have little sense of herself as a separate individual and she may use getting pregnant and having an abortion as a way of expressing these ambivalent conflicting feelings. Becoming pregnant will then be an expression of the non-separation, the similarity, the fusion, and merging with mother, and will also at the same time bring about these regressed symbiotic feelings: 'I am like you – I got pregnant.' In the same way, terminating the pregnancy may be saying to the mother, 'I am not like you. You had me – I am not having this one.' The abortion is a statement that perhaps symbolises gaining a sense of self separate from the mother. Hence the experience of abortion could be a way for a woman to separate from her mother.

The feelings before, during and after having an abortion

Having discussed the internal unconscious level of pregnancy and abortion, I would now like to describe some of the more immediate feelings accompanying this experience.

Feelings when pregnant

Being pregnant is experienced by different women in many different ways. For some, the experience is a very positive one. They like the feeling of fullness; the idea that something inside them is growing; that a part of them has come to fruition. Some, on the other hand, experience it as an invasion which is very frightening. One woman described being pregnant saying: 'I felt as if a monster were growing inside me. I couldn't stand it. I hated the feeling and couldn't wait to get rid of it. I sat and imagined how this monster looked, growing inside me. It was terrible.'

During the few weeks of uncertainty about whether she is pregnant or not, a woman may oscillate between fear, hope and disappointment. When she finally discovers that she is definitely pregnant, many conflicting and ambivalent feelings may come to the surface. The immediate emotion is quite often that of shock, confusion and vulnerability. Sometimes there is a feeling of numbness, quite often a feeling of terror. Predominant feelings may be: 'I wish it were not there'; 'I wish it were taken away by a miracle'; 'I must get rid of it somehow.'

The woman becomes much more aware of her body, feeling vulnerable and sensitive to her environment. Both body sensations and emotions are more available to her. She cries for no particular reason; gets hurt easily; most of the time feels weak and tired. This is a time of emotional turmoil. Even a woman who knows for sure that she cannot, does not want and will not continue the pregnancy often experiences these feelings. Questions like 'Can I?' 'Should I?' 'What is the right thing to do?' constantly disturb her.

In this context, the woman knows that the final decision is in her hands and that whatever she chooses is going to be painful or unacceptable. Things become much more difficult to deal with but somehow she has to get on with doing them, while having to put a lid on the 'volcano' inside. At this stage, the woman is often looking for someone to help her make the decision. The feeling of confusion and helplessness makes it difficult to know clearly what she wants. In this state of ambivalence about the decision, she tends to oscillate from one fantasy to another: each carrying the attractive, pleasant and reassuring, as well as the negative, frightening, rejected aspects of it. From the one fantasy of being a mother and its implications – being tied down, dependent, having demands made upon her, yet loving, being loved, caring and being mature – to the other fantasy of terminating it – to be free, independent, yet losing the love and care, the promise of motherhood. This is a very difficult stage when she needs much support, understanding and acceptance but not advice.

Making a decision to terminate a pregnancy is one of the most difficult decisions a woman has to make. In our daily lives we have to make decisions all the time. Most major life decisions such as getting a job, leaving a job, moving house, etc., could be reversed or changed. Having an abortion, however, is final. It is an absolute decision that cannot be changed or reversed, which is what makes it so powerful and frightening.

Once the decision is made, it is of enormous importance for a woman to know, in detail, how the termination is done: what the physical stages of the operation are, what complications there could be, what dangers or pains could occur, as well as to discuss the emotional turmoil she may expect. A woman who does not get such detailed explanation is often shocked by the intensity of feelings she experiences on coming home, and without knowledge or support is often unable to deal with them. She pushes the feelings aside and gets on with her life. These feelings, however, do not go away and will come up in many disguised ways for a long time afterwards. A woman recently told me she was having some renovations done to her home. For some reason she had to go out to the yard to look at the drains, inside which she saw a dead bird. Having been there for a few days it had no feathers, and therefore looked like a foetus. She dropped everything, ran back into the house and was crying, sobbing and howling for hours, without realising what it was about. After a few hours of crying it became clearer in her mind what the crying was all about. The vision of the bird had sparked off in her mind the feelings she had experienced twenty years earlier.

Emotions after abortion[10]

Having an abortion is often painful in the best of circumstances, but there are some external factors that may operate in an unwanted pregnancy and its termination to make the feelings of loss doubly unbearable and impossible to deal with. These are unnecessary difficulties which could be avoided.

1. Often very little information is given to her about her pregnancy, the termination, the physical or emotional repercussions, and the whole episode is veiled in silence.

2. She is burdened with an internal sense of shame for not being able to go through with the pregnancy. This is confirmed and even increased by her environment; friends, families, hospital staff, who with words or actions may say to her: 'You should be ashamed of yourself.'

3. There is acknowledgment neither on her part nor on that of her helpers of a woman's relationship with a new being growing inside her. In order to feel that she has lost something, she has to acknowledge that she had it in the first place.

4. The fact that she wanted to 'get rid of it' seems to mean she forfeits any sympathy. Why should she feel sadness or loss about something that she wanted to get rid of? On the surface it looks like a contradiction: 'I wanted to get rid of it. Why am I not happy to be rid of it?'

5. The fact that it was her decision which caused the loss often does not allow space for mourning. Since it was her decision she surely has to be courageous and stand by it. She thus has to bear the consequences without grief or mourning.

6. She often feels that she has to punish herself in some way

and that she has no right to feel overtly and directly sad about the abortion.

7. The abortion often is dreamlike: the process is over so quickly that under a full anaesthetic it is difficult to grasp whether the abortion has happened or not.

8. Because of its nature, the termination may become connected with other losses she has experienced in the past, but without the conscious acknowledgment either of this loss or the connection. When I say past loss I don't necessarily mean death. It could, for example, be a parent who left home, or an important relationship with a friend that has ended.

9. The secrecy and non-acknowledgment I have mentioned earlier tends to inhibit the yearning and sadness, and to cause the anger and the guilt to be misdirected. It is usually misdirected on to herself, with blame.

All these factors create a situation where there is no space for a woman to feel the loss, let alone express it and mourn or grieve openly, and will affect the way she feels immediately after coming out of hospital. This will differ for women according to their previous feelings about the abortion and the way in which they have learnt in their lives to go through an episode involving loss. There are, however, three general reactions many women display immediately after an abortion and on coming home from hospital.

Euphoria

Many women will feel euphoric. They will go out a lot, meet friends, feel lighter and happier. They might even be surprised at how easy and smooth it has all been. This is an expression of the feeling of relief and freedom at having solved a problem, having rid themselves of a burden and having executed a decisive action. They will feel strong and in control of their lives. They will feel the need to laugh and have a good time. They will usually keep excessively busy. The feelings of loss, anger and guilt are of no relevance to them in this period. These emotions are bound to come later, sometimes even months or years later, sometimes in a disguised form, apparently with no connection to the abortion.

Detachment

Some women experience a sense of shock or a feeling of inner numbness. They go on with the ordinary activities they are used to doing but with a sense of detachment, distance and unreality. This detachment is an attempt to avoid experiencing the painful feelings connected with the termination. It gives a woman a distance, a non-involved perspective on her environment and her inner world. She may feel an inner emptiness as though what is going on around her is seen through a glass wall. This state may go on for a while. It is not always as strong as I have described.

Depression

Some women get into a state of depression which could be described as a general sense of hopelessness and a diffused feeling of darkness. This state is usually experienced as feeling bad about herself and her life and environment but without actually knowing what it is. At times it comes with the feeling that 'something has taken me over', 'it is all out of my control', accompanied by feelings of worthlessness, emptiness or meaninglessness. Although this state may seem on the surface as appropriate to having had an abortion, in some way it is not dealing with the feeling of loss directly, since the depression is often diffused and not focused or concentrated on the termination.

Some women are able to experience what they have gone through more directly and feel their emotions such as anger, sadness, fear, love and hate. There is, however, no one way that is 'right' of dealing with abortion and no one feeling that is more 'appropriate' than another. What is important is to listen to one's own emotions and try to be with them however difficult it may be.

Anger

Anger is an emotion that is invariably connected to loss. Often a 'normal' response to losing something important, it is directed outwardly with such questions as: 'Why did it happen to me?' 'Why now?' 'Why is life so unfair?' In a termination of pregnancy, there are two factors that make it difficult to direct the anger outwards. Firstly, the abortion itself may be an indirect expression of the woman's initial anger that she was unable to express directly. Secondly, a woman may direct her anger toward the hospital and any inadequacies in the treatment or towards her partner or her family, but her feeling is that ultimately it was her own decision and therefore she is to blame. She feels she was wronged and it is of her own making, hence she misdirects the anger on to herself with self-hate, judgment and blame. She often feels she will be punished and that she deserves to be. Usually, the fear of punishment centres around the fear of not being able to bear children when she really wants to have them.

Guilt

Guilt is sometimes a form of anger directed on to oneself. Many women feel guilty after an abortion. Their guilt can take many forms, centring on difficult areas in the woman's life. Some feel guilty about hurting their mother and father, some about their partner. Some women who were brought up in a religious setting will feel guilty about having committed a sin before God. For some women the guilt is more general or existential and for some it is more specific or personal but in most cases, coupled with the guilt, is a sense of deep shame, of self-accusation and the fear of punishment.

Fear of sexuality

An abortion brings most of the conflicts between motherhood and being a sexual woman into the fore. These conflicts are strongly present throughout the experience of getting pregnant and having an abortion. One common reaction after termination is a fear of sexuality and its consequences. Many women who came to the workshops took some time after the abortion before they relaxed and were able to have sexual relationships again. Another fear of this kind is that of another abortion. I have many times heard the statement, 'I will not go through this experience again.'

Ambivalence

An abortion is an ambivalent action that carries many ambivalent feelings and actions within it. It is saying: 'I want something but I can't have it now.' Or: 'I want something but I don't actually want it.' This ambivalence is, I believe, not only about having a baby. There are many issues in a woman's life about which she feels equally ambivalent but which get 'hooked' on to the one issue of having a baby. It may be a part of herself which she is ambivalent about giving voice to or expressing overtly. The feeling of ambivalence emerges after the abortion in many different ways and it is helpful to look for what the initial ambivalence was about, as well as what the symbols and fantasies attached to the pregnancy and termination mean. For example, a woman who felt ambivalent about her creativity, wanted to study art to create something of herself but was scared of failure on the one hand and of competing with her artist–mother on the other. The abortion came at a crucial time when she had to make a real decision about these things. Her ambivalence about the abortion covered up and diluted the rest. She had to work through these feelings to get at her initial ambivalence about creativity.

Envy

Women often feel envious after a termination, envious of other women who have babies. At times they will walk through the streets looking at babies in prams and feel very sad. Some women cannot bear to visit friends who have newborn babies, as it is too painful to be with them.

These are all relevant feelings. There are no correct ones that one 'should' feel. It is important, however, to have enough time after the abortion to look at what one's feelings and conflicts are, to be able to feel the loss, sadness, relief, lightness, etc., without believing that one is 'obliged' to feel one or another.

Some positive aspects of abortion

An abortion, painful and destructive as it may seem, is not always just a negative experience. Some women have expressed the positive aspects of pregnancy and termination even though the pain, sadness, and negative aspects exist as well. For example, for some women, the experience of pregnancy was exhilarating. Becoming pregnant in spite of the wish not to have the child constituted an important event for them. To feel something had been created inside and was growing within them, without the actual need to carry it further and have a dependent baby, was very meaningful. One woman felt that what she wanted was the creative aspect of it, the sensation of being pregnant. Many women had feared they were infertile so that getting pregnant was an affirmation of their fertility, proof that they were able to conceive, which was important since so much emphasis is put on being fertile in our society. Connected to that is the feeling of wanting to 'try out' being a woman.

Some women have a feeling of power and being in control in a life where they often feel powerless and out of control. For some women this was the only time in their lives when they allowed themselves to be irresponsible. Ordinarily they felt they had to be punctual, responsible, do everything the right way, and somehow they felt trapped by always being tied to the rules and having to be perfect. Being irresponsible was a different experience for them.

Making an important decision was another aspect that was a new experience for some women who felt their lives were for the most part dictated by others. For some women, the act meant, on a symbolic level, a statement of separation from the mother and becoming an individual, a woman with her own power.

It is clear that the price to be paid in a case of termination of pregnancy, emotional and otherwise, is enormously high and none of the positive aspects that I have mentioned would outweigh this; but it is important not to ignore these aspects.

Men and abortion

The issue of abortion not only touches very deeply the women who have had an abortion, but also women who have never had one, and even men. This may be one of the reasons why it is such a taboo subject. The issues it brings up include questions of life and death; women's and men's roles in society; questions of power and control; the power of reproduction in women and men's fear and envy of it. It brings up the issue of being unwanted and the potential rejection that each one of us ponders on at some point of our lives. 'Was I wanted?' 'How did I come into this world, this family?' It brings up many existential queries from time to time. Each one of us has strong feelings concerning motherhood lurking somewhere. As well as these issues, there are important aspects of pregnancy and termination which, in my opinion, affect a man's attitude towards his partner. The first one is men's fear of women's ability to reproduce. This brings up many feelings for the man as the 'potential' father: the fear of control, the power, the self-sufficiency that women sometimes feel when they become pregnant; the fact that, in the end, it is a woman's decision, and hers alone. Staying with a woman who is pregnant by him seems to some men the utmost commitment and some may find this daunting. On the other hand, staying with a woman who has an abortion may feel like a rejection of himself in some way. Either way, men find the experience of abortion very difficult and threatening. This is the reason why this experience is a 'make or break' issue in many relationships.

Sometimes a man supports a woman fully, goes with her to

the hospital, gives her space, safety and encouragement to talk about what she feels, accepts the anger she is expressing and generally supports her during and after the experience. For many women, however, the reality is quite the opposite. Often the man cannot cope with the strain and leaves. Often, he doesn't want to know, and the woman is then left with having to deal on her own with two losses at the same time: the loss of her pregnancy and the loss of her relationship, involving pain, anger, sadness, and despair.

Men often feel a sense of loss, guilt, anger, and lack of control about the decision. These feelings are difficult for many men to express or even acknowledge, both because of their conditioning in our society and because the experience is 'at one remove'.

Both because abortion is so strong a taboo and so contrary to social concepts of what it means to be a 'woman', *and* because it involves so many painful, unconscious feelings, women need a chance to talk about it, free from any preconceived notions about what their feelings/reactions, etc., 'should' be. What needs to happen is that the taboo should be broken to give a chance to more women to talk to each other about their abortions and attendant feelings. Women should be allowed to have and express whatever feelings arise in them and not feel obliged to have any specific set of feelings. In talking about the experience of abortion more women should aim to understand the conflicts underlying it. Abortion should become, rather than an experience unnoticed, denied, unimportant, one that is easy and immediate to talk about.

This article is dedicated to Jeanette and Rami, my parents, with love.

And acknowledgments are due to my friends Sue Krzowski, Shoshana Simons and Margaret Green for their love and support. To Liz Greene for helping me realise so much. To Jose Nicholson for the title and a lot more. To Marilyn Senf who co-ran the post-abortion workshops with me at the beginning.

Mira Dana

Notes

1. Information on the political campaign (in this and the following pages) came out of a discussion with Julia Goodwin, Natalie Petinaud and Gwenith Donovan from Women's Reproductive Rights.
2. Mary Daly, 'Beyond God the father – towards a philosophy of Women's Liberation', quoted in Adrienne Rich, *Of Woman Born: motherhood as experience and institution*, Virago, London, 1977, p.266.
3. Adrienne Rich, *Of Woman Born*, p.266.
4. ibid., p.267.
5. Eileen Fairweather, 'The feelings behind the slogans', *Spare Rib*, Issue 94, p.27.
6. Adrienne Rich, op. cit., p.34.
7. Luise Eichenbaum and Susie Orbach, *Outside In ... Inside Out*, Penguin, Harmondsworth, 1982, p.84.
8. Jean Baker Miller, *Towards a New Psychology of Women*, Penguin, Harmondsworth, 1976, p.131.
9. Dionora Pines, 'The relevance of psychic developments to pregnancy and abortion', *International Journal of Psychoanalysis* 63 (3), 1982.
10. In this section I draw on Bowlby's ideas. See John Bowlby, *Attachment and Loss*, vol. III, Penguin, Harmondsworth, 1980.

7
Women in the oppressor role: white racism

Introduction

In this paper I will be exploring what happens when white women come together in groups or workshops to work on racism. From the emotional work done in these, it becomes evident that experiences of oppression in early childhood provide the fertile ground in which the unconscious roots of racism develop and are allowed to flourish. The common factor linking the many and varied experiences of oppression is the conscious and unconscious abuse of power in relation to children.

Some of the papers in this book explore a part of this dynamic although they do not use these terms to describe it. They focus on the position of one of these unconscious abusers, i.e. the mother in the mother–daughter relationship, placing her in the context of her own oppression and powerlessness. This paper has a similar aim, in that it explores what lies behind the conscious and unconscious abuse by white people of black people.

Although we still have a long way to go in eradicating both the unconscious and socio-economic elements of racism, various political movements have attempted to come to grips with the internal as well as the broader political manifestations of oppression. After World War II, Third World struggles against colonialism began to achieve substantial victories. In their wake came a growing understanding and analysis of the internal struggle which had to be waged to throw off the shackles which colonialism had exerted on the minds of the colonised. Although the external struggle has been won all over the planet, the psychological battle, complicated by the inroads made by imperialism, is still in progress. Inspired by these events, the writings of Frantz Fanon[1] and by liberation leaders closer to home, the colonised peoples living in the United States started developing a black consciousness movement in the mid-60s. 'Black is beautiful', 'black pride', 'black power' were the war-cries. This was a battle for people's minds.

Through the following decade, an understanding of how external events and their accumulated internal repercussions combine to keep people oppressed continued to develop, as did an awareness of the importance of the psychological sphere in bringing about political change. These ideas were taken up afresh by women, giving the movement for women's liberation a new impetus. They have since informed other movements for the liberation of oppressed peoples, such as the gay and lesbian movements, anti-psychiatry, and the campaigns by people with disabilities. So these theories about the internalisation of oppression have become part of our shared awareness and it is difficult to remember today that certain phenomena which this concept enables us to understand appeared very puzzling twenty years ago. We didn't really know why giving women the vote didn't change their position in society, or why black children given equal educational opportunities didn't do better in school, or why many oppressed people ruin their lives with alcohol and other drugs.

So we have begun to learn about the psychological factors that work against political change, the conditioning which appears to keep us on the side of the status quo. In the early years of the Chinese revolution, for instance, this problem was recognised and addressed by holding criticism/self-criticism groups at the workplace and within communities.

It has proved much harder for progressive movements to acknowledge the internal factors at work in creating the oppressor. We tend to explain oppression in terms of external forces – economic power, tyrannical dictators, totalitarianism. Many sociological theories have been advanced to try to explain how it is possible that masses of people can be mobilised to collude in oppressing others. Psychodynamic studies have explored sadism, violence and racism.[2]

The way we have dealt historically with oppressive behaviour does not make much sense. We have idolised and voted for it. Then, when we've seen that it doesn't work and the perpetrators have fallen from grace, we have hounded them, held trials, called in firing squads, used imprisonment, torture and 'short sharp shocks'. This is very much the same treatment that is meted out to the oppressed when they attempt to act more powerfully.

However, in recent years, groups and courses have developed in an attempt to tackle the interplay of social and personal factors which contribute to the conditioning of people in the oppressor role, for example men against sexism, racism awareness training. The work (called 'unlearning racism') that I am concerned with here is another development in this category. It includes the understanding that many oppressive attitudes and behaviours are rooted in the unconscious and cannot simply be eradicated by rational argument; that people need support and encouragement as well as correct information if they are to give up firmly held oppressive convictions. One of the assumptions of this work is that people *will* do so if such support and information are provided in a respectful manner.

A number of projects for training in racism awareness have emerged in recent years. They vary in approach and are different from unlearning racism.[3] There is an increasing demand for these as more black people enter employment in job categories where there were none before and put pressure on their organisations. Community groups have also pressurised London borough councils and the GLC so that funding bodies now require from voluntary organisations the implementation of an equal opportunities policy as a prerequisite for obtaining funds. Personal attitudes with regard to race are also explored in local authority job categories and an anti-racist stance has become a criterion for obtaining a job in these instances. As a result, many organisations are seeking anti-racist training. But, although racism awareness training courses profess to address feelings involved in 'personal' racism, they do not appear to be wholly successful because at the outset they do not allow space for the oppression people experience in relation to learning and perceiving reality.

Various critiques of racism awareness training have been published recently. Some attack what they see as a therapeutic approach to what should be a political struggle,[4] and others the lack of a sound theoretical base to most racism awareness courses.[5] I agree with some of the arguments raised, the main one being that the priority now is to change racist institutions. Another criticism is that the 'personal' racism carried by white people is their own problem, and does not necessarily concern others. However, as a white person and as someone interested in the psychology of human relations, I am necessarily concerned with both issues. Since oppressiveness, like oppression, is manifest on both levels, the individual and the social, I feel it is important to explore the theme in terms of early object relationships – these being our first experiences of a culture in which we learn to be both human and inhuman.

I am a South African Jew born during World War II. I never felt there was much of a role for me as a white in the struggle against racism – you could do something fairly minor and end up in prison for it – so, like many others, I left the country. But I have always wondered whether there were not in fact more choices available.

I was living in the United States during the early days of the current wave of struggle for women's liberation. I had never thought of myself as oppressed in any way while living in South Africa. I had ascribed my isolation and misery to the fact that I felt responsible for what was happening. It was a relief to get out. The early ideas of the women's liberation movement were very compelling to me. I felt they explained a lot about other women's lives but I still did not see how they applied to me. As a Jewish woman, I grew up having the same opportunities as my brothers and was expected to be tough, assertive, educated and intelligent. (The fact that at the same time I was supposed to be 'feminine' and unthreatening to men only struck me later as paradoxical.) After joining a consciousness-raising group on coming to England in 1970, I became interested in the role of conditioning in shaping our thoughts and ideas about ourselves and the way we behave.

This interest led me to try out various forms of therapy and eventually to train as a psychotherapist. It was, however, only when people I knew and trusted started exploring their oppression as Jews and Jewish women that I began to identify more and realised that some of my early unhappiness could be explained in terms of being oppressed (an issue I explore more generally later in this chapter).

I was always aware, however, of my role as an oppressor with regard to racism, and was looking continually for some way of dealing with whatever was preventing me from committing myself more fully to the struggle against racism. What follows in this paper is in a sense my attempt to answer that problem. I went to a short workshop in the United States led by Ricky Sherover-Marcuse[6] in which her main point was that whites are hurt by racism – not in the same way as are people of colour, but nevertheless, for most of us, the quality of our lives is seriously reduced by it. I knew this to be true for myself, and I eagerly attended as many of her classes as I could. Much of the theory presented here derives from her thinking and writing; the examples come mostly from my own experience of leading unlearning racism courses in London.

I am using the term 'racism' to mean black/white racism, although who is black and who is white is not always clear. I am aware that other forms of oppression are also referred to as racism, for example the oppression of Jews, of the Irish, of 'foreigners' – Cypriots, Spaniards, Turks, Italians or Latin Americans. I do not refer to these as racism in this paper. I am also aware that the terms 'black' and 'white' represent peoples of many different cultures, religions, languages, histories and geographical locations. Racism and colonialism have made it difficult for us to recognise this rich variety of differences on both sides of the black/white divide.

Some of the theory on which this work is based will become evident from reading the following sections, but some basic assumptions, developed further at the end of the chapter, need to be stated.

Nobody is born racist, or wanting to be racist. Racism is institutionalised in our society and every white, as well as every black person, has therefore been affected by it, has 'learnt' in various ways to be racist. This is not their individual fault. The reason why racism on an individual level is hard to face is because it is painful to do so. The roots of this pain are largely repressed and unconscious; they lie in the confusions that result from having been lied to and misinformed by people we trusted; and in the pain of having tried unsuccessfully to resist the 'learning' of racism. We are born with the capacity to be aggressive if wronged in some way. 'Unlearning' racism therefore involves the expression of this repressed pain, for example by talking, laughing, crying, trembling and storming about.

The best way for white people to examine the racism they carry is in 'whites only' groups; equally, the best way for people of colour to explore how they have been oppressed and to gain solidarity, is in various groupings of Third World people. This is parallel to the need, in dealing with gender oppression, for separate men's and women's groups. We have discovered many reasons why separate groups counteract our conditioning and prove empowering. Perhaps the most important here is that a white person's acquired racist conditioning is a black person's oppression. Safety is not enhanced by repeating racist situations as they exist in society. There is a point in informing each other but only when people have dealt with their feelings separately, sufficiently to be able to listen.

Great progress can be made towards removing the clamp that racism exerts on the minds of white people by work of this kind. It can contribute to improving conditions so that whites and people of colour can lead more fulfilling lives. However, since racism is a social and institutional problem, it cannot be eradicated without radical transformations in our institutions and class structure as a whole.

The workshops on which this chapter is based were often held at the Women's Therapy Centre, and this context is important. People assumed that emotional explorations were on the agenda. Although the participation was extremely varied in terms of class, nationality, ethnicity and sexual preference, because of the way the workshops were advertised the women who came were all white. Frequently I co-led classes with a Jewish working-class woman. This enabled any lone Jewish participant to feel somewhat safer and therefore to feel freer emotionally. My being a white South African was also helpful, not only for the safety it provided to any South Africans or people with colonial backgrounds who might attend, but because it served the purpose, as it does in the wider society, of alleviating liberal guilt. Whereas in Britain today I do not consider it useful for liberals unconsciously to dump their own feelings about racism on individual white South Africans, in a workshop setting this allows for the opening up of other deeper feelings.

In what follows I will delineate the presenting problems and issues that people bring to the unlearning racism classes and workshops that I have led, and I will describe how I have worked with some of them. The examples cover a broad spectrum of personal experiences with racism rather than an in-depth examination of one or two clients, or of ways to deal with institutional racism. I will then present some of the ways in which these workshops have proved useful and indicate some ways forward. Lastly I will look at some theoretical considerations about oppression in general and the oppression of young people in particular.

At this point, I feel it necessary to say something to the many people who have attended my workshops and classes and to whom I implicitly promised confidentiality. The examples that follow are mostly drawn from my own workshops. I have taken great care to see that no one is identifiable – except perhaps to someone who was actually there at the time. However, I apologise if anyone reading this feels they are being misrepresented in any way. I trust that most people who have been to my workshops feel that the approach is important and should be more widely used and that this chapter is a first step in making the work more publicly known. I have been most moved by people's openness with me and I therefore hope that nothing written here will prove to be an abuse of that trust.

Working with white racism

Curiosity

In a safe and structured environment people begin to remember their early feelings of power and curiosity and some of the particular moments when they first became confused by misinformation they received and, as a result, reluctant to question further. For instance, as adults, white people are aware only that they're afraid to ask things they don't know about other people, such as asking Afro-Caribbeans about their home islands or Muslims about their religion. They think they ought to know but somehow they don't.

Some examples people did manage to remember from childhood will help to illustrate what happens. One woman remembered how as a child she had gone with her grandmother to market. She saw a black man and she asked her grandmother why he was black. Her grandmother replied, 'because he's covered in chocolate'. Knowing that that couldn't be true and not wanting to tell her grandmother she was a liar, she pursued it. She asked, 'Could I go and lick him then?' at which point her grandmother became rather angry and uncomfortable and pulled her off in another direction. In this case the little girl, dependent on a good relationship with her grandmother, blamed the tension between them on the black man. It was his fault that her grandmother got cross, therefore he was 'bad'.

The way liberalism masks or denies differences appears equally irrational to a child. For instance, a little girl growing up in an area where there were very few black people, herself very blonde and blue-eyed, was standing in a supermarket queue. Her mother, a propos of nothing, volunteered to her the information that the man standing behind her was no different from her and she should remember that. One look was sufficient to verify that her mother must have been seeing things very strangely that day. The only possible inference for her was that black people made her mother behave in a very bizarre fashion. One might feel somewhat daunted (as this child did) at the prospect of questioning any further.

Misinformation

We seldom realise how painful it is to receive misinformation. Because it is painful it becomes stuck in our minds in a way that is different from relaxed learning.

A woman from a city in the Midlands came to a workshop. As an adult, she had always lived in mixed neighbourhoods and although she acknowledged there were tensions, she enjoyed it, had friends from other cultures and so on. However, since she'd had her first child, she'd become particularly scared of the black people in the neighbourhood and very worried for the safety of her child. She was thinking of moving out to the suburbs and was feeling very guilty about her fears, knowing they were racist. It emerged that she remembered sitting on her grandmother's knee being read to from a story book. It was about black people in Africa being cannibals and eating white babies. With this memory came feelings of fear and she realised the origin of at least some of her fears for her baby.

Often what contributes even more to the hurtfulness of misinformation is that we received it from people we loved and admired, parents and teachers. Frequently we don't remember anything in particular; we are filled with a sense of conflict and confusion as we try to explore these early experiences.

Resistance

Childhood relationships with black people don't always exist on the level of curiosity, misinformation, 'areas you mustn't walk in' or 'children you mustn't play with', although for many British adults, these seem to be the main features of their experience.

In the United States, South Africa and India, white people experienced daily confrontations with racism, and those who grew up in these countries carry considerable guilt about how much they have colluded with racism. South African whites, in particular, are held up as being the worst examples of racism and many will accept this view of themselves. Some have embraced with relief the more liberal attitudes to Third World people that other countries allow. They will seldom acknowledge, however, nor will anyone else let them, that the tensions of living in their homeland must have been fairly unbearable for them to have willingly given up legally entrenched white privilege. They come bravely to workshops, expecting to be attacked and feeling that they deserve it. The acknowledgment that they too, and not only black people, have been hurt by growing up with racism provides them with a view of their experience they've usually never had. Such a different slant makes memories more accessible because the accustomed defences one mobilises against blame are unnecessary.

It begins to emerge particularly dramatically for these women, that as children many of them resisted the injustices at home. Some can remember asking questions about the strange discrepancies in their homes. Why was it that a black woman they felt so close to wasn't in fact a member of the family, couldn't eat at the same table, had to use different cups and plates from the rest of the family? Questions such as these were responded to by lies, stone-walling, ridicule, anger or even beatings. It was often very difficult for a child to ask parents such things – there was a lot at risk. Many learnt early who it was who had the power in these situations and that per- haps it was best to stay quiet and not rock the boat.

The questions may be remembered but usually the conse- quences I've described are not recalled as easily. They take some working through because the results of asking such ques- tions were often traumatic – as is also the case for the other uncomfortable questions children frequently ask, for example about sex.

Projection

The projecting of one particular form of personal or collective distress on to other situations or people is a common tragedy in the history of racism. Situations in which black people are the victims of white distress have occurred repeatedly within the personal and public spheres in many families, on farms and in factories in almost every country in the world. Because racism has been so deeply rooted in the collective unconscious of whites for many centuries, black people become the convenient scapegoats of our unconscious fears. This, for instance, happened to a male client in psychotherapy. He was physically quite small and myths which exaggerate black physical prowess and sexuality made him fearful of black men. His guilt at his desire for closeness with his mother and his fears of castration at the hands of his father, were so unbearable that they led him as a child to acts of self-inflicted physical punishment. As an adult he was extremely scared of walking past black men in the street – his fear of castration was projected on to them.

Recent emotions as well as those from childhood can be projected on to black people. One woman described how she was becoming short-tempered with the black women who came to the clinic where she worked. She was less tolerant with them. In encouraging her to let rip at these absent women, it became clear that what was bothering her was the frequency of their pregnancies and the number of their children. She had been wanting to have a child for about a year and had not conceived. She realised how envious she was of the supposedly greater fertility of black women, and understood better the source of her current difficulties with them.

Black people are also 'used' by whites as 'good' objects on which to project feelings of idealisation, admiration, sexuality etc. Often the important factor here is their non-whiteness. Whiteness can mean one's family and community and if associations with these are extremely painful one may wish to escape. Black people may provide one with this possibility. This is most likely to be the case for a person who has grown up in a family community which exhibited racism quite overtly. A white child may wish to disavow her family and community.

As an adult she may surround herself with black friends and lovers or be working together with black people in liberation struggles. There is nothing intrinsically wrong with this if it is done from a sense of pride and rootedness in one's own community, but in this case it may be a reaction to shame, self-hatred and despair, none of which makes for good alliance. Of course the mechanism is not unusual in the history of any individual – we are frequently splitting and using people as objects as a way of dealing with the feelings which we don't want to acknowledge.

Why people come

People have often partially transcended what was originally instilled in them before they come to a workshop. An awareness of certain feelings has brought them to this point. That in itself is a stage beyond the irrational acting out and harassment which one witnesses in buses, streets, schools, on housing estates, etc.

Many of the white women who come to unlearning racism workshops are workers in the caring professions; they are students, social workers, community workers, teachers, nurses, midwives. They work with Afro-Caribbean and Asian people and they realise they have been affected by racism. These women feel the need to grapple with the task of changing what is unconscious and internalised with regard to racism. As feminists many of them have faced similar issues with regard to their own oppression as women. They are consequently a little more prepared than other women to acknowledge how oppressive they are in turn to black and brown people.

But it isn't only because of work that white women come into these workshops. Some women have intimate relationships with black men or women or their own or adopted children, and have had the courage to admit that they are having difficulties in these relationships. Others can't handle the racism or anti-semitism of their parents. Some feel filled with shame and can't admit to the kinds of relationships they had, growing up as children of colonial administrators, with servants. In all these examples there is the beginning of an awareness that even as a white one has been damaged by racism.

Once there is an awareness of wrongdoing or injustice, most people feel guilty and responsible. They see themselves as hurtful, not hurt. This is a recipe for remaining stuck and may be the main reason people often have to be coerced to hold or go to racism awareness courses at work.

Safety

How does one create a safe situation in which we can own up to the thoughts, often a source of great guilt, which we hold deep in our minds?

In individual or group psychotherapy, there is a structure by which one or two people take responsibility to contain the situation and the feelings. My workshops are led and structured to allow for only minimal discussion at first. Because feelings surrounding racism are so strong, people are only too prone to attack each other or feed each other's feelings of hopelessness about how difficult it is to tackle institutions, when what they need to be doing is tackling themselves. So the exercises and questions are designed for each person to focus on her own feelings and experiences. As a leader, I try to show other members of the group by my own example what we should be doing – listening respectfully and with acceptance, rather than giving advice, criticising or judging. I also prevent group members from intruding or commenting on each other.

Emotional work is done in groups of white people for reasons of safety. Even in a different context, for example mixed (black/white) work groups, I would present mainly a theoretical understanding of what's going on to the whole group, as opposed to working emotionally with them. As we have learnt with men and women, it reinforces the oppression to re-create a situation in which the people targeted by the oppression are forced to be supportive or to listen to non-target people. These terms – target and non-target – [7] may be unfamiliar to the reader. I use them because it is important to have words which don't have the emotional content associated with 'victim' and 'oppressor'.

❧

Innocence

Communicating the belief that people are not to blame for the oppressive role they play, that they would never willingly choose it, is crucial to counteract in some measure the guilt which people bring to classes. You may disagree with this belief but its importance as a working assumption has been proved over and over again as people cease feeling so culpable, stop rehearsing their guilt and are freed to explore their underlying feelings. For example, as black people feel their strength and solidarity, whites are more often confronted about being racist. Women who have experienced these encounters sometimes present a guilty defensiveness. If I assert that they are innocent, that they do not mean to be racist (as I do in my initial talk), welling up from underneath the guilt is tremendous rage at what these women perceived as an unjustified attack on themselves by black people. The confrontations had triggered off feelings about other oppressive attacks they had experienced and were powerless to handle at the time – sometimes because they mistakenly believed they had invited these. This was what happened for at least two rape victims who attended workshops.

It is a common assertion that people have a stake in their privilege, be it parental, male or white, and will not surrender it. In theory I assume that when white people realise the extent of their hurts from racism, they will readily relinquish their stake in it. In practice, however, the evidence suggests that people's fears stop them from risking any upheavals on an institutional level. Paul Scott writing as Daphne Manners in *The Jewel in the Crown* about the role of two colonial administrators in an Indian town, says:

> They were predictable people, predictable because they worked for the robot. What the robot said they would also

say, what the robot did they would also do, and what the robot believed was what they believed because people like them had fed that belief into it. And they would always be right so long as the robot worked, because the robot was the standard of rightness. There was no originating passion in them. Whatever they felt that was original would die the moment it came into conflict with what the robot was geared to feel.[8]

So what I am in effect saying to people is, 'You had original feelings, thoughts and ideas. You expressed them many times in different ways as children. Something has happened to you to make you lose your courage. We will take a look to see what that is.' This works because largely it is true. I do not ask people to explore all the times they went along with institution-alised racism and continue to do so. I go into the reasons for this more fully under the heading of 'Guilt'.

Unexpected changes of focus

The most interesting feature of emotional work on being racist is that hardly anyone ever sticks to the topic, unless they have been working in the arena of oppression for many years. This is of grave concern to many workshop participants who have come feeling puzzled, confused and guilty about themselves and hoping to find a simple answer. They feel they have not tackled the subject and will blame me for not leading them there. Nevertheless, if one attempts to work with any one of them they will invariably revert to the hurts related to their own oppression.

Recently, during a weekend seminar held at the Women's Therapy Centre for women in the caring professions, I led a two-hour supervision group on the topic 'Working with women from different cultures'. I suggested they talk in pairs for a short time about where they were having problems and then pick a specific situation. I then asked some of them to volunteer to work on that situation with me. All three who volunteered chose as their problem situation one in which they were inter-acting with men of different cultures, not women. Nobody even noticed this was happening. They all chose sexist situa-tions in which they were the victims to some extent – thereby confusing the issues. Now why did this happen? I think it is both inevitable and necessary.

These women were in a women's group. What they had in common was their oppression as women. The greatest emo-tional safety lay in working on that. Few of us ever finish with the hurts we've endured as a result of sexist conditioning. At the precise moment at which these women were looking to change their oppressive attitudes they were unconsciously revealing the source of them within their own oppression. In the presence of black people such behaviour is oppressive because it is a denial of the reality of how racism assaults them. However, it is often difficult, though of course not impossible, to examine oneself in the non-target role when one is still carrying so many feelings about being targeted.

In any case, these are all routes to the same distress. The first woman talked about how difficult she found it to wel-come and befriend new immigrants (in this case the male head of a family) who came into the advice centre where she worked. There was at first a lot of talk about how he had misinterpreted her behaviour, seen it as sexually inviting and so on. Here she confused her own hurt as a woman with her discomfort about classism and racism. I suggested she imagine I was this man and she try to do what she felt she'd failed to do at the time. She couldn't, she said, because I was not a man. So I suggested she try welcoming me. As a Jew and a foreigner I could never have enough of it, I explained, and besides, no one had ever welcomed me to England anyway. She tried. She was extremely timid and tentative. I asked if she had ever been made to feel welcome. She burst into tears; no, of course she hadn't. There was no warmth for her in her family; she had always felt unwanted. After some minutes of her crying and saying what it was like, I suggested that she try welcoming me again. And this time there was much more warmth and confidence in her voice and gestures. Everyone in the room noticed the difference.

I cannot overstress the point that working on one's own oppression, particularly oppression as a child, is an essential precondition for any individual changes with regard to racism. On the other hand, there is no necessity for me to stress it in a group because, given sufficient safety, most people will do it anyway in such a setting.

A Jewish male intellectual shamefacedly admitted that he thought black people were stupid. Within a few minutes he was shaking and crying about how his survival had depended on him being clever, that to be considered stupid was a constant source of terror although he had always feared that he might be. He could never relax about it the way black people appeared to him to be able to do. A common feature of oppression of Jews is the belief and sometimes the reality that survival depends on academic achievement.

A whole group began, over a series of classes, to view every suggestion and intervention I made as that of an authoritarian teacher. Their role as oppressors was completely overlaid by their feelings of being targeted in the classroom. There were hoots and shrieks of delight when finally one of the 'pupils' pushed me back to my seat. They were releasing tensions from childhood to do with being oppressed at school.

This phenomenon has been labelled 'denial', that is, the oppressors are denying responsibility for their role. But this overlooks an important dimension – one of my assumptions is that no one would ever willingly choose to take on the role of oppressor if they themselves had not been systematically oppressed. If one imagines a person on a see-saw alternating between the two possibilities, oppressor and victim, then emotional work on either role undermines the fulcrum and eventually the whole structure will collapse. This is particularly true of the ways we have unconsciously internalised oppression.

Another way to tackle some of the distress is to explore the target and non-target roles that exist within a group of whites in relation to other forms of oppression prevalent in society such as classism, anti-semitism, anti-Irish feeling, to name but a few. In one class, my co-leader and I (both of us Jews) set aside time for 'all you ever wanted to know about Jews but were afraid to ask'. Most were too embarrassed to come out with the misinformation we'd hoped to hear like 'Do you have horns?' or 'Are all Jews rich?' They were very tentative and careful, an example of what has happened to so many of us. Our natural childhood curiosity about differences appears to have been destroyed. As the atmosphere became more relaxed and we cracked jokes and didn't attack anyone, some people began to feel safe enough to be curious and to ask questions which were much more important to them. So, although Jewish oppression is not the same as racism (there being different historical and class issues as well as stereotypes), this opportunity encouraged people to push beyond their embarrassment to give vent to curiosity about differences.

There are other important reasons to explore the different backgrounds within the group. Firstly, you cannot be proud of other cultures and delight in their richness if you are not proud of your own. By 'proud' I don't mean the defensiveness which hides feelings of shame and inferiority and I don't mean that one doesn't question certain aspects of one's culture. A sense of one's own rich roots is however essential if one is to meet on an equal level with a person from a different background. Perhaps this is self-evident, but anything short of it allows for a situation which can be filled with humiliation, envy, contempt and denigration.

Another reason is that by having each person examine her background it usually becomes abundantly clear that we are both oppressors and oppressed – we carry both roles. Any group of white women are oppressors in terms of racism, the oppressed in terms of sexism. The existence of both roles within ourselves, and the concomitant social implications, form an area insufficiently explored, where the external world impinges on internal psychology. It is the internalisation of our personal experiences of oppression which perhaps cause us to feel inadequate, ugly, ridiculous, invalidated, objectified, fearful or terrified. If these experiences remain unresolved, we then project on to the external world. Who or what we perceive as embodying a threat to our existence, be it personal, social or economic, is very much determined by institutionalised prejudice and prevailing myths and stereotypes which serve to manipulate and fuel our fears. It could be black people, but it could equally be AIDS (and by inference any gay man), the IRA (and by inference any Irish person), terrorists and Communists (anyone fighting for national liberation), and so on. Our neuroses feed the institutions, and the way oppression is institutionalised feeds our neuroses.

Many people develop a way of thinking about institutionalised oppression as a hierarchy of who is most victimised in society. Hierarchies of social power, however, don't translate exactly into personal experience. We think of men as less victimised than women. Some would say they are not victimised at all. Nevertheless, little boys feel powerless too. To deal with these feelings they are provided with toys, stories, images and heroes. These differ from what is offered to little girls, who feel equally powerless. Belonging to the gender that is supposed to carry the guns may generate fear rather than a sense of power. For instance, I worked once with a man who had recently been appointed to his local Community Relations Council. This was his ostensible reason for coming to this particular short workshop. He admitted he was particularly frightened of groups of black youths. As we explored why and he shook violently in my arms, he remembered stories and films from his youth which depicted lonely forts in the furthest reaches of the Empire in which a few whites stood fast against hordes of advancing natives. From these 'learning' experiences he had determined never to go to Africa as it was far too dangerous. 'But', he said in a very scared young voice, 'now Africa has come to us!' I never explored why this man had a particular identification with the imperial army or British colonial administrations but one can assume that many English men over forty-five might have had. It is striking how much misinformation was contained in the images he had. Who in the larger context was frightened of whom? Who really had the power? Why were whites depicted as the victims rather than the victimisers?

Since I have only rarely worked with men in these classes I found the work with this man particularly revealing. I doubt that any woman would ever have identified, in her childhood, with a lonely fort-holder of the Empire. Part of male conditioning is being expected to have to fight for one's country, perhaps to die. This is not a feature of female conditioning. The closest I came to sensing the connections between colonialism and racism on an individual emotional level with women had to do with how they felt about the pink 'colonial' areas on pre-1960 maps, or the memories some had of 'owning' and naming a black child in Africa at school, encouraged in the 1950s by missionary societies.

Isolation

One feature of oppression experienced in childhood is the feeling of isolation which, as it were, goes along with the invalidation. If, for instance, I ask women to imagine themselves as the only white person in a particular situation, a large variety of imagined experience will be shared. Some common features will be fear, shyness, not wanting to be there and, in particular, not feeling welcome. If I then work with this feeling of what it would be like to be fully welcomed into a black person's life, home and family, a woman will have a tiny glimpse into the patterns of isolation she carries with her all the time. Let us say she is a woman from a working-class background in the north of England, come to study in the south and who has made friends with black people in college. She will probably add that actually she feels even more unwelcome with southern English white people, that is, that the isolation is something she has felt ever since she left home. I expect if we had longer, we would find the feelings of aloneness go even deeper.

With so little opportunity to discharge these feelings except in close relationships, we will re-experience them in almost any situation in which we have been made to feel, or feel ourselves to be different. In the group the distress will be associated with being from a different background from the others, but its roots may go back to being the fat girl in class, or the one who spoke with a different accent or never had any friends, or even further back, to never really feeling loved by one's mother.

Remembering the battles

I have already mentioned that everyone as a youngster tried to fight against the lies, misinformation and injustice they per- ceived around them. However, it is extremely hard for people to recognise that they did and in any case we define fighting in a particular way. We exclude the struggle involved in knowing some adult action is wrong, and asking about it, or choosing to read certain books in an attempt to find out the truth. We think of fighting simply as confrontation. Of course many children were not so intimidated and have tried actively con- fronting adults too.

Although for many people these memories may take a lot of work to bring to light, sometimes they can emerge dramatic- ally within the first couple of hours of a class. For example, at the end of the first class of a series, the participants engaged in a short discussion about cultural differences and how a liberal education often encourages one not to notice them. A white South African woman in the class began to get vehement. She claimed that she saw no difference between Irish and English people for instance, and more importantly that there was absolutely no difference between black people and white people. This raised a storm in the other group members. In London today such statements and thinking are considered racist. But she wouldn't budge. I realised suddenly – probably because I am also a South African – that she was expressing herself at a different level of human interaction and, what is more, that some distress was locked up in her refusal to con- sider what the others were saying.

I quietened the others, insisting that her background was different and differences were what we were there to notice and asked them to pay attention. I told her to continue speak- ing as she had been. Within half a minute it became clear she was locked into an incident that happened when she was four years old. It was about her beloved black maid having to use a different toilet from the rest of the family. She had objected and shouted as she was doing now (over twenty years later) that the maid was no different from them and why did she have to use a different toilet and different crockery, and so on.

She did not win that battle. Because of it she had been rigidly fighting ever since. No matter how much it caused her to be labelled racist in England in 1983, she knew with the certainty of a four-year-old that she was right and her mother wrong and that she was fighting *against* racism and not continuing to be racist as everyone in her group was alleging.

In the context of South Africa in which black people are treated as less than human, she was right. Despite ethnic, cultural and some minor physical differences, people with dark skins are not a different species from people with pale skins – we are all part of the human race. However, this event in the class reveals another important issue. If we carry around painful memories of resisting and losing – evidence of one's powerlessness as a child – we are not always able to behave appropriately in the new situations we find ourselves in; we can only fight old battles. We are helpless in this, as this woman was, unless we can locate the hurt and discharge it. Otherwise we are liable to confuse a group of white women in 1983 in London with an English mother colluding with racism in 1960 in South Africa.

Remembering the resistance, that one is not intrinsically a 'bad' person, is therefore an important step in lifting the heavy burden of guilt. Realising why one lost and remembering the victories, all serve to direct one towards regaining a sense of individual power. This is the major prerequisite for fighting institutionalised racism, or any oppression, including one's own.

One of the major painful consequences of the many forgotten battles is the splitting up of families because of racism. Many people live thousands of miles away from their families so as not to encounter the racism they exhibit. Siblings do not speak to each other. It is a major area of unfinished business within countless white family relationships. It is usually within the family that one had to confront one's own powerlessness and impotence to change a situation that one knew was wrong. So those feelings are re-experienced when one meets up with them. Many sons and daughters choose to make these occasions as rare as possible.

A fair proportion of people coming to workshops and

classes feel themselves to be 'not very racist', and want to know how to confront people who are 'really racist'. The situations in which they feel they need help vary from arguing with parents and siblings over dinner, to witnessing whites being abusive or violent to people of colour. They find themselves responding by shouting, walking out of the room, by a feeling of paralysis or terror.

In working on this, I will remind the person of my basic assumption – that they are human beings not wishing to be racist – and encourage them to replay the situation as powerfully as possible. For women, this involves role-playing actions which cut deep into areas of women's oppression – being assertive, developing a deep and frightening growl as opposed to whining or complaining, maintaining confidence in one's own thinking in the face of ridicule or invalidation and in one's ability to defend oneself physically, refusing to step down and adopt the position of victim, and so on. Practising in a workshop and overcoming the inhibiting feelings equips one to deal more flexibly when the situation arises again.

Handling racism also requires developing further the talents which women are conditioned to acquire – to listen carefully despite not liking what you hear in order to glean the 'kernel of truth' in what the person is saying. If you listen carefully, people will always tell you where they are hurting, that is, why they are racist. I encourage class members to listen to each other in this way.

Guilt

White women work readily in the ways I've described. It is much harder to tackle guilt directly. One does it mostly by working on the ways one has been oppressed, eroding the whole structure (the distress pattern) from underneath. Beavering away at the foundations will eventually topple the structure. From my own experience this takes many years.

I have not worked with many people who are ready to explore usefully how they've colluded with racism. Largely what lies behind the guilt is tremendous grief and it doesn't help for a person to relate a story of how she let herself and other people down unless she can get in touch with the feelings of grief by doing so. So I will use myself as an example in this section.

While leading classes, I realised I was having a particular difficulty in dealing with the sexual objectification that white women project on to black men, that is that they are 'studs'. I understand the roots of it as being in our oppression as women with its emphasis on sexual objectification and the way this focuses our feelings on to our bodies, combined with believing the racist misinformation that abounds on this subject. But that didn't help. I felt quite disgusted at this particular form of distress and found myself being judgmental. Someone suggested I ask myself, 'Is it true what they say about black men?' I knew of course what they did say – these things are common western misinformation. 'Surely I don't think this stuff?' I wondered. I didn't know.

When I was given attention by a white man with whom I felt completely safe (a rare occurrence), the feelings and thoughts I'd stored up over many classes and workshops came tumbling out in sequence. I had had my own history with some black men. Almost all of it was occluded or unconnected in my mind because almost all of it was very positive. This was painful too, given that I grew up in a place where one was taught not to notice black men and particularly not to notice that they were men.

Male servants were the first men I was close to and who paid attention to me on a day-to-day basis. My father and uncles were much more remote. I'm sure one of the domestic servants was the first man I was sexually curious about. The first adult male I ever saw naked was when I was seventeen and was assigned a half-share of a corpse in the dissecting room of an anatomy laboratory. He was black.

The first man I ever really loved and felt loved by was a black fellow-student at university – a fact never acknowledged by me before because I was not allowed such feelings. They were forbidden. I released great floods of grief about this, mostly at not having had the courage to act on my feelings.

If there is a single reason for my doing this work it has to do with what I consider to be my lack of courage at that time and my desire to repair the damage my blindness did to him by not recognising the importance of the relationship. I have since realised that this was also damage done to me. Different of course from how he was hurt, but hurtful to me none the less.

Gains so far

People realise their guilt is a waste of time. The workshops direct people towards looking at early experience. They realise that it is in their *own* interests to do emotional work on racism; that the issues of lack of assertiveness, of fear, envy, guilt are hurts that they need to explore for themselves. Because certain feelings are split off and unconsciously contained as racism, coming to one of these classes may be the first time a person is put in touch with certain negative feelings. This is important for the integration of one's personality. People are often quite shocked by the intensity of the feelings involved and are pushed into a realisation of how much work there is to be done. Some people, as a result of coming to a class or even a short workshop, look for ways to continue exploring their history, for example through therapy, co-counselling, etc.

Many people realise their ignorance, and recognise the importance of gaining knowledge and taking pride in their own backgrounds. They may see the hurts of classism or anti-semitism as being more significant in their childhoods than the hurts of racism. They may feel the need to deal with these emotionally as well. In some instances, self-help anti-racism groups have continued after the classes.

A sense is gained of the significance of lack of respect to *any* person. With the understanding that the theory provides, stopping such behaviour does not appear such a daunting task as most people would think. There is often a sense of empowerment to *do* things.

For women coming to these classes there is often a great deal of initial anger at the thought of men being viewed similarly to whites as the non-target group in relation to sexism. There is considerable difficulty in imagining the ways in which men have been hurt by sexism; even if this is acknowledged, it is considered trivial. (I expect any black person reading this will feel the same way.) Usually by the end of a class in which this has been a theme, there is much greater understanding of the non-target role especially in relation to men.

There is usually a dawning realisation that being an ally to a person of colour involves knowing a great deal about one's own background, remembering with pride one's own history of resisting injustice as well as one's participation in the history of racism. It involves being able to listen and tolerate the differences between people, expecting to make mistakes, knowing that people of colour will be angry with you to the point of what appears to be unreasonableness, and learning to take it. It involves also knowing that people who view you as an oppressor may try to mistreat you – but this you need never accept.

You may wish that you could learn enthusiastically about other cultures, make friends boldly, gaily take risks and make mistakes from time to time, stand up to racist behaviour with confidence and be a splendid ally, rejoicing in how safe you have made it for your black friends to become angry instead of careful around you. Perhaps you have some excellent proposals for dealing with racism in your workplace that you would like to feel assertive enough to put over well? Even if you only want to act in one of these ways, you may find that you still fail. Feelings of powerlessness defeat our best intentions. There is an almost universal acceptance that there's not much one person can do. This is not reality. The reason we feel this way needs to be explored further.

The oppression of young people and the interlinking of oppressions

Racism is promulgated and perpetuated by all the institutions in our society, by the circulation of myths and misinformation, and more often and more insidiously by lack of information and ignorance of that lack. It affects both how we view our history and all our plans for the future. This is only made possible by the interplay between social forces and individual susceptibilities.

Our susceptibility to absorbing racist ideas and theories has one major root cause, also institutionalised in society but not always recognised as such – the oppression of children and young people and the resultant sense of powerlessness inculcated in them at an early age. Most of the examples in the previous section corroborate this, but as psychotherapists we are so used to seeing early distress as individualised expressions of hurts perpetrated within a particular family, that we are in danger of missing the wood by concentrating on the trees – that is, forgetting the institutionalised components of early distress. Child-rearing has had many more books written about it by adults than, let us say, the education of black people has had by well-meaning whites. We only have to look at all the many and varied theories that have been presented as scientific fact over the last forty years to realise how riddled with myths and misinformation child-rearing is. As with black people, we have seldom let children speak for themselves. This might seem reasonable, because we are led to believe that for the first two or three years they cannot do so. However, any parent is aware that in those early years children are quite capable of communicating their needs and desires. Nevertheless they have often been denied their feelings, experience, sexuality and self-definition; as with any oppressed group.

Many adults today were treated when children no better than laboratory animals if they were hospitalised, were given less recognition and comfort than pets at home and have experienced schools as places of invalidation, if not incarceration. This is not so much due to adult viciousness as adult ignorance.

One of the most telling examples of the oppression of young people has been over the question of incest and sexual abuse. The enormity of this situation for children is just beginning to be discovered.[9] One of the reasons it has been hidden for so long has been that children were not believed even when they actually tried to tell someone. The prevailing myths within the adult world about children are that they make things up, that they should be seen and not heard, that if you 'indulge' them they will 'get spoilt', and that it was, and still is, perfectly acceptable for adults to assert their power by violence.

As psychotherapists, we see the individual casualties of adult ignorance, misinformation, invalidation, violence, neglect and disbelief. We do not blame the individual mother but we encourage our clients to express their anger at their own mothers. In ordinary life, however, try as a parent to let your child carry on crying on a bus, or pee in a public place or even try breastfeeding beyond the first year or two. You will be criticised, ridiculed and made to feel extremely isolated. Our culture has institutionalised the oppression of children.

So children accumulate hurtful experiences – abandonments, deprivation, times of confusion and powerlessness. Loving attention and the expression and containment of painful feelings will enable a child to deal with and recover from many of these. But frequently these outlets are not available to a youngster. Even if there is loving attention, a parent may not be able to tolerate a child's full expression of embarrassment, shame, anger, fear or grief. Few adults (when it was their turn) were allowed such a release of their tensions. So more often than not traumas are stored and eventually repressed. But that is not the end of the story. Sooner or later, the stored-up tensions become unbearable and the incident is re-enacted in some way (repetition compulsion in psychoanalytic terms). Taking on the role of the person who did the hurting is one common method of re-enactment.

Particular social roles reinforce and encourage re-enactment. The most striking example of this is all the customs and rituals surrounding the fag system at boys' public schools. Young boys systematically mistreated when they first enter the school are then encouraged in their senior years to repeat exactly what was done to them. This was the perfect training ground for the colonial administrator who would be expected to treat his Third World underling with similar contempt. The role provides the opportunity, and the person filling it experiences enhanced social status, a sense of self-worth which contradicts his early experience, and at the same time a release of tension which accompanies the re-enactment of a hurt in a position of greater power.

Certain roles institutionalised in society have their own momentum. Teachers will say how they never intended to treat children 'that way'. But they find themselves shouting, for example, or about to use violence. They may begin to see themselves pitted *against* the children rather than as the allies and collaborators they had always intended to be. Of course, there is hardly anyone alive today who has not experienced some form of mistreatment at school. Being in the position of teacher sanctions the re-enactment of childhood hurts. There are for instance schools where corporal punishment is still allowed. If that is the case, then lesser everyday crimes like invalidation, ridicule and humiliation, and the suppression of creativity will surely go unnoticed.

I am deeply indebted to the Swiss psychoanalyst Alice Miller[10] for exploring the common situations of childhood with such sensitivity and uncovering the 'poison' in universally accepted adult behaviour. She does it particularly effectively in the case of Hitler[11] who is often cited as the one person who must be an exception to the theory that there is a causal relationship between early victimisations and adult aggression. He is thought of as an aberration – the incarnation of pure evil. However, not everyone mistreated or abused as a child goes on to treat their own children or others in the same way.

The more suppressed the expression of any outrage, the more split off the hurt becomes. Hatred for the perpetrator is not allowed so it is repressed, stored and internalised until such time as it has some outlet, such as the socially sanctioned forms of hatred as racism, classism, anti-semitism and misogyny. If one has the opportunity to find oneself in a position of greater social power than others, the hatred may be actually lived out. The form of the abuse, mistreatment or violence is often perpetrated in exactly the way it was originally experienced. Victims become oppressors, beaten children become battering adults, invalidated girls become critical mothers, childhood poverty and deprivation produces adults unwilling to share resources with 'foreigners', concentration camp survivors may behave sadistically towards their children.

Filling a certain role in the structure of our society may push one inevitably into acting as the willing or unwilling agent of a particular oppression. The roles of factory manager, trade union official, policeman, TV producer, hospital consultant, staff nurse, psychotherapist, teacher, social worker, husband, mother, place people potentially in positions of authority over others. Anyone in such a position is exposed to the possibility of becoming an agent of oppression. I would like to introduce a way of describing these social roles which neutralises the attacking aspects involved in labelling someone an 'oppressor', an anti-semite, a racist, a male chauvinist – the implication being that that individual person is evil and enjoys being oppressive rather than (which is more often the case) being the unwilling, rather ignorant, powerless agent of a particular oppression. This is not to say that sadism and greed do not exist – that there are not occasions on which the perpetrator apparently enjoys his/her viciousness and violence. There are definite secondary gains for repeating hurts done to oneself in the position of the perpetrator; as Alice Miller says: 'Those who persecute others are warding off knowledge of their own fate as victims.' Greed (the desire for social status, money, power, fame) fuelled by the way our societies are organised, allowing privileges only to the chosen few, acts as an additional motive for maintaining whatever status we have managed to achieve, be it in relation to class, race, or gender. These feelings push us into taking on, where possible, the role of agent of the oppression rather than the victim.

In the following diagrams I use the terms 'target' and 'non-target' to describe the relationship of members of different groups to a particular oppression, for example, white women are the targets of sexism, but are non-target in relation to racism.

If we look at racism in particular, the *non-target* group are whites – the agents in oppressing people of colour, who are the *targets* of racism.

People of colour react in various ways to being targeted.

Diagram 1

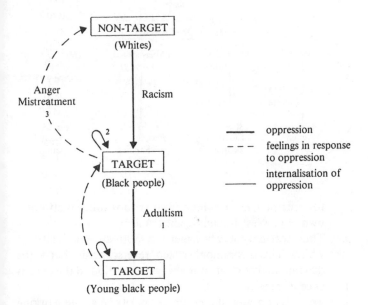

These fall broadly into three categories.

1. For example, if they are lucky enough to grow up and have children, that is, if racism does not kill them off too soon, they may find themselves inadvertently passing the hurt on to young people, filling the role as agents of adultism.

2a. The target group may *internalise* the invalidation and lack of recognition they have experienced, thinking badly of themselves, possibly believing themselves to be what the stereotypes say they are. On the other hand some will attempt to be themselves while at the same time trying to skirt the stereotypes and non-target definitions of who they are – an exhausting process which can lead members of target groups in general to numb themselves with alcohol, drugs and depression.

2b. Target group members often hate others in their own group who seem to fit the stereotypes more readily. In the case of racism, the internalised racism may also be directed

Diagram 2

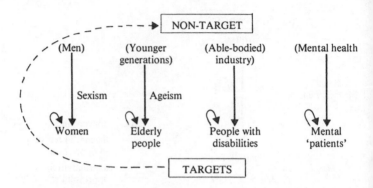

towards people of colour from groups other than one's own, e.g. West Indians against Asians.

3.   There will inevitably be anger and mistreatment directed at whites. This is commonly called 'reverse racism' but as the diagram makes clear, it is always in reaction to the experience of racism.

If we focus on any one group in society, e.g. the working class, and look more closely at this group so as to include a few

Diagram 3

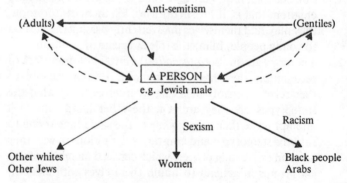

other forms of oppression, such as sexism and ageism, we get Diagram 2. This does not mean that sexism and ageism are the only forms of oppression. The whole list would take many pages . . .

This is an oppressive society. Every person in it is, or has been, a member of both target and non-target groups.

We can then examine what an individual white person attending an unlearning racism workshop brings with her in terms of target and non-target experience. In this case, I will choose for convenience an able-bodied, middle-class, heterosexual young Jewish male from an Ashkenazi background (i.e. European).

He would have been targeted as a Jew and as a young person growing up. He may say that he personally has never experienced anti-semitism. He would in this case be denying or numbing the pain he has experienced in knowing that anti-semitism exists in the world and in his own country, and in knowing about the accumulated hurts in the history of his people. Fears of extermination may still haunt him even if he was born years after World War II. Similarly, anger and fear at how British imperialism caused evictions and starvation may haunt and gnaw at an Irishwoman who has grown up in England and experienced neither. History is very important in shaping one's particular experience of being targeted: the history of slavery still intimately affects every Afro-Caribbean person's view of themselves.*

The young Jew may have been hurt by both Jewish and gentile adults when he was a youngster. He will probably be a good deal more in touch with these experiences. He may well have responded with anger and indignation to both these forms of oppression, but no matter how encouraging, proud and nurturant his upbringing was, he would be hard put not to have internalised some aspects of the attacks he undoubtedly experienced. The very thing that brands him as a Jew – circumcision – would constitute one of the earliest attacks. But even without considering all the consequences of that, living in an

---

* It is not only the target group that is affected. Try thinking of explaining slavery to a young white child you know or imagine teaching a lesson on the extermination of the Jews in a German classroom. It is no wonder people avoid doing it. I have seen a whole roomful of English people in tears as an Irishman expressed his rage and grief at the events of Bloody Sunday. Outrages perpetrated against anyone are painful to all of us. Given the opportunity (watching the news on television can hardly be considered one of these), we will feel it. Mostly we find it unbearable to be aware of so much pain so our vision narrows, we can only see what we can bear to see.

environment which circulates negative myths and stereotypes about Jews will constitute a possible source of self-hatred.

The bad news is that if he is currently not obviously hating himself or other Jews, he will probably be projecting his hatred on to groups with less social power than himself, for example women, or black people or children. How much he does of one rather than another will depend on many factors which include his particular experiences of oppression, his capacity to identify and his ability and openness to learn from the environment.

The good news is that emotional work done to transform self-hatred, shame and powerlessness in oneself, reduces the need to project these feelings on to other people. This is the main *emotional* work that needs to be done to fight racism, that is, contradicting by intention, action and release of feelings the internalisation of powerlessness. It is, of course, not the whole story in the fight against ignorance and *institutionalised* racism. Nevertheless any action taken to reverse the oppressive processes in society which select certain groups for targeting and then isolate them from others, requires the assertive challenging of authority both internally and externally.

What one does with one's regained power is not my brief in this paper. But it would involve co-operating with others to raise awareness of the key issues in a particular institution, to organise priorities, exercise leadership, provide support when the going gets rough and to meet and consult with the black and Third World groups or organisations that are involved, bearing in mind that in certain situations being powerful may mean encouraging, acknowledging and allowing for black leadership to take over because it is the most appropriate way forward. At the same time one would also have to ensure that such skills are sufficiently valued that there will be other jobs for anyone who is able to be so effective.

Acknowledgments

The difficulties for me in the writing of this chapter were much alleviated by the support of my niece Sharla Green-Kibel, who read the manuscript and helped devise the diagrams on my visits to Cape Town, and Armourer Wason, who rescued me at a crucial time and, in the middle of her own exams, came and wrote down what I said while I talked aloud.

Margaret Green

Notes

1. Frantz Fanon, *The Wretched of the Earth*, Pelican, Harmondsworth, 1983.
2. Morton Schatzman, *Soul Murder*, Penguin, Harmondsworth, 1976; Alice Miller, *For Your Own Good — hidden cruelty in child-rearing and the roots of violence*, Faber & Faber, London, 1983.
3. Antoinette Satow, 'Racism awareness training; training to make a difference' in Ashok Ohri (ed.), *Community Work and Racism*, Routledge & Kegan Paul, London, 1982, ch. 4, pp.34-42; Basil Manning and Ashok Ohri, 'Racism — the responses of community work' in Ohri *et al.*, op. cit., ch. 1.
4. A. Sivanandan, 'RAT and the degradation of black struggle', *Race and Class*, 20(4), 1985, pp.1-33.
5. Ahmed Gurnah, 'The politics of racism awareness training', *Critical Social Policy*, no. 11, 1984, pp.6-20.
6. Ricky Sherover-Marcuse, *Issues in Co-operation and Power*, no. 7, 1981, pp.14-15; Sherover-Marcuse, *Present Time*, Rational Island Publishers, no. 44, July 1981, pp.36-37.
7. Ricky Sherover-Marcuse, *Present Time*, Rational Island Publishers, no. 47, April 1982, pp.3-6.
8. Paul Scott, *The Jewel in the Crown*, Panther, London, 1973, p.551.
9. Alice Miller, *Thou Shalt Not Be Aware — society's betrayal of the child*, Pluto Press, London, 1985.
10. Alice Miller, *The Drama of the Gifted Child and the Search for the True Self*, Faber & Faber, London, 1983. Also *For Your Own Good* and *Thou Shalt Not Be Aware*.
11. Alice Miller, *For Your Own Good*.

8
Change in women

> ... love me a little,
> ... just a very little,
> as you would love a baby.
> It's all that I ask for.[1]

This article explores and compares three books concerned with the question of the link between the individual and society, with women particularly in view. They are *The Rocking of the Cradle: and the Ruling of the World* (1976) by Dorothy Dinnerstein;[2] *Outside In . . . Inside Out* by Luise Eichenbaum and Susie Orbach;[3] and *Psychoanalysis and Feminism* by Juliet Mitchell.[4] Each of these texts has drawn on psychoanalysis in an attempt to articulate the link between the individual and society. Each uses a different theoretical framework both for the individual and society.

Since the resurgence of feminism in the mid to late 1960s certain sections of the women's movement have been highly critical of psychoanalysis. It was thought that the aim of psychoanalysis was for the analysand to become better accommodated to society; and that one of the consequences of this was a blunting of political awareness. That was supposedly the outcome of the different power positions occupied by the analyst and analysand which made the analysand highly susceptible to the analyst's assumptions and values. From the early 1970s onwards there has been a reassessment of psychoanalysis, and various women writers have drawn on different psychoanalytic theories in attempts to clarify women's sexuality and position in society. Feminism addresses many questions to external reality, with a view to changing it. What we as women have gradually become aware of is that our attempts to make changes are to some extent subverted by forces within ourselves that resist change. Psychoanalysis is a way of exploring the various explanations of these resistances.

Psychoanalysis is a set of clinical practices which offers people à path to knowledge and self-understanding as a way of relieving mental and emotional distress. It is also a collection of theories about the processes and structures of the human mind and how it functions. At the heart of this is a question about the nature of human beings: about the limits and possibilities for change, in our links with society. These questions pose ethical problems which in the main have been considered the domain of religion, politics and sociology. Much recent psychoanalysis has failed to acknowledge such questions. It is no coincidence that it was initially feminists who reintroduced psychoanalysis into the political arena. This led at first to an opposition to psychoanalysis and later to a reassessment of it: a reassessment which is still continuing. Feminism is concerned with the limits and possibilities for change, and psychoanalysis has an important contribution to make in this arena.

This article is intended to clarify some questions by comparing three different theoretical approaches. The comparison is between the three texts listed above, and not any other writings that these authors may have produced and which might modify the positions held there.

The Rocking of the Cradle: and the Ruling of the World

Dinnerstein makes problematic the relation between the individual and society. There is a dissonance between the two which stems from our internal understanding of ourselves in the world, which has been unable to keep pace with external change and development. She argues that this dissonance is sustained by our present-day system of sexual arrangements. These sexual arrangements in which women 'rock the cradle' and men 'rule the world' are derived from the early history of civilisation when they were necessary for the survival of society. Human beings' capacity for understanding and knowledge was elementary. Women spent the major part of their adult lives pregnant or lactating. Therefore it had to be the men who went out into the wider world hunting for food, etc., while the women took responsibility for the care of infants and young children, preparation of food, etc. This division of labour, originating in an external necessity, has become through the centuries so deeply ingrained that it appeared to many – as it still does to some – as immutable. However, argues Dinnerstein, our knowledge and control over our lives have changed and grown so that such sexual arrangements are no longer necessary. For example, birth control methods mean that biological differences need no longer determine how men and women pursue their lives. Not only need not, but they *must* not. The sexual polarisation of men and women's activities is not only no longer necessary, it is also highly dangerous. We are driving ourselves towards the possible extinction of the species. The use of technological knowledge for devastating purposes is evidence for this.

Inner psychological reality has not kept pace with external social possibilities, because inner psychological patterns developed over the centuries are very resistant to change. And, she continues, a strain that has grown over the centuries has now reached crisis point. Our present outmoded sexual arrangements are sustained by a tacit collusion between men and women. At the basis of this collusion is a denial of death and human mortality. The denial has its origins in a characteristic peculiar to the human species: prematurity of birth followed by a prolonged infancy. Because of its prematurity the baby is for a long time after its birth unutterably dependent upon another to take care of it, if it is to survive; and its subsequent process of growth and development is very extended. At first, because of this absolute dependency, the infant necessarily experiences the mother as being one with itself. This illusion is at the root of life. The infant starts out from an experience of an oceanic feeling in which there is no differentiation and only gradually has to discover itself as a separate human being with an 'I'. The pain experienced as a result of this process of separation is equivalent to our later understanding of death.

Development, for Dinnerstein, occurs through dis-illusion and the discovery of not being one with another. Out of this evolves another human characteristic – that of pleasure in enterprise:

> the pleasure of enterprise, of mastery – through which (as Freud points out) each member of our species tries, while at the same time harbouring deep misgivings about the value of the effort, to console itself for a peculiarly human loss – the loss of infant oneness with the world – and to assert itself against a peculiarly human discovery – that the most important features of existence elude control.[5]

Growth and development are then always deeply ambivalent experiences, since there is always an underlying wish to return to an illusory state of oneness. The child consoles itself for its primary loss as it explores the difference between self and other, by developing its capacity for mastery: 'the exercise of competence and will'.[6] What it discovers is that

> as it starts to affirm itself as a wilful, enterprising 'I', ... its body, precious vehicle of the 'I', is also the 'I' 's hateful jailer and saboteur: through the body the 'I' learns how puny it is in the face of inanimate obstacles; how limited its power is to make what it wants happen; and most humbling of all, how deeply it can be forced to knuckle under to another, alien, will. The later discovery that flesh is transient and will finally cut the 'I' off from the world resonates with this earlier discovery of the flesh's treachery, made as the 'I' first starts to form itself.[7]

Under the prevailing sexual arrangements we use our capacity for mastery to deny the pain of our mortality and of the loss of our archaic unity. The loss is renounced rather than mourned. If it were mourned then it could be retained as an experience to enrich our lives.

Men and women renounce this loss in different ways. Men develop a capacity for mastery in a form which enables them to deny the body, and therefore, for Dinnerstein, deny their emotional pain and 'early delight in the vulnerable body's joy', with 'a compulsive concentration of attention and energy on that which can be predicted, controlled, manipulated, possessed and preserved, piled up and counted.'[8] This form of mastery is derived from our mastery over our anal functions and is a transformation of them. It is eminently suited to present-day society outside the family. Taken to an extreme, it leads men to deny their mortality by attempting to impose their will on nature, and by failing to accept that there are always things beyond human control.

Women's relation to their bodies, argues Dinnerstein, is inevitably more active. Their physical attributes, particularly menstruation and childbearing imply that women cannot deny their bodies in the same way as men can. They are also in daily bodily contact with the children they bring up. What follows for Dinnerstein is that women in certain respects are more emotionally aware than men. None the less, women still deny loss. They do so by closing themselves to life beyond the family net. They are thus able to deny the pain of loss of their archaic oneness by absorbing themselves in family life, and not developing their capacity for mastery further. The consequence, for Dinnerstein, of such a difference between men and women is that the two major components of social life – the 'rocking of the cradle' and the 'ruling of the world' – are segregated at a time when they need to become integrated.

Men collude in this denial of loss because they can directly satisfy their desire to return to a merger with the mother in their sexual relations with women. They can also vent their archaic rage at this loss through relationships with women. Under the prevailing sexual arrangements flesh is either glorified or debased. Women come to represent the 'dirty goddess' at whom men alternatively direct rage and grief, but whom they do not mourn.

Women collude in sustaining themselves as the primary care-takers because, firstly, they derive power from the emotional tie that develops between mother and child, and this can be used in their relationships with men. Secondly, because they can obtain relief for their own wish to return to the original experience of unity, by mothering their own infant. Thirdly, because to change position and to become a member of society who directly – rather than indirectly – influences the path of history, means tolerating doubt. To undertake this sort of work means living with a question as to the value of the effort, as well as risking failure. By remaining within the circle of the family, women can avoid these doubts. Fourthly,

> Man's hungry, worshipping enjoyment of her body, his dependence on her presence and on her comforting physical services, allow her to relive vicariously through him her own old love of the maternal flesh and her own old, luxurious dependence on physical care, while he relives his directly. His contempt for and cruelty to her body allow her to relive directly, with masochistic pleasure, the fleshy humiliation that both endured as infants, while he relives it vicariously through her.[9]

In this situation the woman identifies with her own mother and thus is party to the attack, identifying as she does with the aggressor.

Dinnerstein's analysis in which men and women unconsciously collude with each other 'is not a conspiracy imposed by bad, physically strong and mobile men on good, physically weak and burdened women. Male rule has grown out of biotechnological conditions which we are just now, as a species surmounting, and out of the psychological impulses that inevitably develop under these conditions.'[10] The collusion is breaking down because of biotechnical developments and this has brought closer to the surface of human beings a primordial rage and grief against the mother for loss of oneness. It is not possible for women to bear the brunt of these emotions. Women can no longer continue to represent both for their children and for men all that is emotionally invested in this early contact when the child experienced itself as one with the world. Dinnerstein believes that we must mourn this archaic loss if we are even to find a satisfactory form of social life. As things stand our capacity for enterprise is being misused and has become lethal. Men have the power to rule and therefore to destroy the world with women's tacit agreement.

The basis of Dinnerstein's analysis is found in the account she gives of human mental life, and the process by which babies develop into adults. She thinks that human beings are stuck in an infantile, pre-verbal stage of emotional development, and that if our adult potential is to be released we must understand the basis of this stuckness. It is important, therefore, to explore the major components of Dinnerstein's developmental theory.

Dinnerstein's baby is born prematurely into the world. This baby's basic emotional need is for a feeling of oneness, and it can experience this because of the mother's *emotional tie* to her infant. Since this experience of unity is a necessity for the baby to begin to be able to order its experience, it is in a sense enslaved to its mother. Dinnerstein's baby is a passionate baby – a mass of feelings and sensations, both pleasurable and unpleasurable, which have to be ordered if the baby is to fulfil its task of developing into an adult human being with a faculty of reason. Since the mother is generally the primary caretaker it is her task to order these powerful sensations and experiences through caring for the baby's physical and emotional needs and through naming them. She inducts it into a relation with itself and others. She carries it inside her; gives birth to it; and then in intimate contact with her – mind and body – the baby begins to be able to sustain the enigmatic journey of giving meaning to its life and understanding its connectedness with society, and the temporary nature of its existence.

For Dinnerstein the foundation of human reason is built upon the way in which the baby deals with the presence and absence of the mother. However, the baby's capacity to experience this is also determined by the mother's capacity to manage the archaic feelings re-evoked in her. The infant's initial grasp and understanding of itself is constructed through what Dinnerstein calls the 'will' or 'intentionality' of the mother. She gives value and meaning to the infant's body, its emotions, its first sounds, etc. She orders the infant's experiences with her oohs and aahs, dos and don'ts, good and bad, etc. When she is there in her all-providing capacity the mother is experienced as wonderful and good but in her absence she can only be monstrous and bad. The infant, therefore, is subject to another's will long before it has a will of its own. Its own will – its own subjectivity – is developed through the will of the mother. This initial experience the infant has with the mother will mark all its future relations with others and the environment.

Because the infant's first experiences of being loved, cared for and comprehended is with a woman, the infant, whether boy or girl, makes an initial primary identification with woman. This not a sexual identification nor is it an identification with a human being as such. It is an identification with something more akin to God. Something that is all-powerful and all-providing. It is both wonderful and monstrous. As the baby becomes aware of the absence of the mother – specifically the feeding mother-breast – it gradually acquires an awareness of a lack of unity. The gradual disillusion that such a unity exists introduces the baby to the problem of how to make sense of this lack, and this predicament leads it to develop a capacity for reason. It is here that Dinnerstein's account becomes problematic.

Dinnerstein draws heavily on the work of Melanie Klein, particularly her paper 'Envy and gratitude'.[11] I have drawn on this paper directly rather than on Dinnerstein's account because Klein's assumptions underlie Dinnerstein's work. Klein studied the inner mental life of children, and constructed a theory about the origins and processes of mental life. Her work has an instinctual basis to it. She believes, for example, that the conflict between love and hate is innate, as is 'the infant's innate feeling that there exists outside him something that will give him all he needs and desires'.[12] Klein argues that these innate processes are the outcome of the infant's inevitable experiences while developing in the womb. In other words she argues not for a biological basis to mental processes as such, but that mental differentiation begins to occur prior to birth: it is these very first experiences from conception to the first half year of life that order our mental life. The infant is thus born with the seeds of a moral sense, which is founded in the desire to protect that which it loves – at first the breast that nourishes it. This leads Klein to develop a theory of splitting in which the infant protects this goodness, which is both inside and outside, by splitting it off from the bad. For it can only feel good about itself to the extent that it can protect itself from feeling that it has destroyed the good, external object. The external environment can exacerbate or modify these internal processes.

The problem with this position is that ultimately meaning is determined – an inevitable outcome of a bodily experience. This stands in contrast to Mitchell's account of Freud, showing that meaning is always constructed retrospectively. Such a theory as Dinnerstein's assumes that our experience of external reality can be distinguished absolutely from our internal fantasies – that we can make a clear separation between inner and outer, if we are fully able to mourn. Meaning is derived from the infant's direct experience of its body. However, what is missing is *how* meaning is transmitted from the external world to the inner psychological world. For Klein, all that the mother can do is to create an environment in which experiences already pre-structured can be integrated internally, and perhaps named. Questions of morality and ethics are already answered and need no further development, since moral life is located in the desire to protect the loved object.

What is useful for us as feminists in these ideas is that the mother cannot be held entirely responsible, as she often has been, for the infant's predicament. The infant brings into the world with it these innate feelings, some of which are likely to be stronger than others and for that nobody can be blamed. The strength of its instinctual life is something that every child has to struggle with for itself.

The father in Dinnerstein and Klein is accorded a very secondary position. In Dinnerstein, the father has little effect on the infant's mental life until the child can perceive him. In this sense she is an empiricist: the unconscious is structured through empirical experience. Since in the early months the infant has little direct experience of the father, his place in the infant's mental life is of less importance. By the time the child is able to perceive him, the child will have a greater sense of otherness, and so the father will appear more human and less all-powerful than the mother. His authority, therefore, being perceived as relatively limited, brings relief. He becomes subject to the child's curiosity as the capacity for reason develops and the search for the 'I' progresses. The father is seen to go outside the home and do something else. He is perceived as a 'participant in history' and the child's understanding of the wider world is intimately connected with the father's activities. Sexual difference then becomes understood in terms of these differential activities of the parents.

In Dinnerstein's view, the major differences between the sexes arise from the fact that women have prime responsibility for childcare, although biological differences do intervene in emotional life (as we shall see). It is this division of labour in present sexual arrangements which disadvantages the little girl. The little girl, if she is to be heterosexual, has to change the object of her love from mother to father. Heterosexuality is the dominant social demand, but Dinnerstein also sees an instinctual tendency towards it. This change of object inflames her rivalry with and jealousy of the little boy, since he does not have to renounce his mother in this way. This is Dinnerstein's explanation for penis envy, which she sees as a social phenomenon. It has to be asked here why certain things are selected to be regarded as innate, in order to explain others which are not. The little girl's, and later on the woman's, homosexual feelings are also more disadvantaged, because they are marked by this early archaic experience of oneness with the mother, without the compensating feature of an experience of difference.

At puberty the girl's body intervenes in her emotional life with physiological changes – developing breasts, menstruation, etc. – and she experiences her body in a new way. In Dinnerstein's view, there is a sense in which the woman's body is more present than is the man's; a woman is less likely to lose touch with her bodily experiences and tends to be more emotionally aware than men. Her capacities for menstruation and for bearing children combine in giving her a relation to her body and flesh which men can evade in themselves.

Little boys are advantaged because they can retain their original love object, their mother, and as they become aware of the father, can experience a means by which they can break away from the maternal emotional tie. A boy can enter the external world of history. Dinnerstein also thinks that the boy's, and later on the man's homosexual feelings are less complex since the father is perceived as a separate human being by the time he becomes the object of the boy's love. The little boy is eager to follow in his father's footsteps and be able to grow into a man. Since, for Dinnerstein, a man's relation to his body is less active, his emotional life is also likely to be less active and women come to embody everything he finds painful in himself. He is then free, she thinks, to go out into the world and develop his capacity for mastery. On the other hand in lovemaking he is potentially returned to the original state of oneness with mother. So his relation with women is extremely ambivalent. For the woman, the man is less likely to enable her to make an emotional return to this original state, because his body is physically so different from a woman's; so her way of satisfying this archaic wish takes a more indirect route via mothering and becoming the 'scape-goat idol'. In either case, she renounces the possibility of affecting directly the making of history.

Outside In . . . Inside Out

The question central to Eichenbaum's and Orbach's project is 'how society makes a woman a second class citizen'.[13] This question came out of their political concerns, as feminists who were very heavily influenced by the American women's liberation movement. The movement – particularly in the States, but also in some groupings here in Britain – was originally very opposed to psychoanalysis, both its theories and practices. They criticised it for reinforcing the very values and cultural norms that they sought to undermine and change. These criticisms were levelled at psychoanalytic writings on female sexuality in particular, with Freud seen as the worst culprit. The movement also criticised orthodox analysis for failing to understand the place of the external social and political world in psychological understanding. They thought that this was sustained by a form of practice which supported the analyst as an omnipotent figure, who knows all in relation to the patient, and to whom it seemed that the patient had to submit. In their view, the analyst took a position of power and authority similar to that of many medical practitioners and other professional workers. This authoritarian stance encouraged a passive and childlike acceptance of the analyst, which they believed subverted the patient's desire for autonomy and self-determination. They argued that this was particularly true for women since it re-created a woman's experience, without creating the possibilities for change. Another criticism, made in Britain at least, was that psychoanalysis was only considered appropriate for educated people, i.e., the middle class, and that it was not generally available on the NHS.

Eichenbaum and Orbach established the WTC with these criticisms of psychoanalysis very much in mind, but although they agreed with a lot of the criticisms, they also agreed with those who argued that psychoanalytic theory had something to offer. They were also considerably influenced by a lot of work that had been done in the States, work that addressed questions to the mother–daughter relationship and sexual differences in general. They wanted to develop a practice which would be based on a more equal footing between therapist and client, while at the same time taking into account a woman's experience of herself as 'second-class'. They were also searching for a form of practice which could account for the internalisation into mental life of the external, social world, and particularly the social values that it accorded women. What came to be called 'feminist therapy' was a way of tackling these questions. (It may be interesting to note that at the Women's Therapy Centre there are those who call themselves feminist therapists, and those therapists who are also feminists.)

The aspect of therapy that Eichenbaum and Orbach think distinguishes feminist therapy from other analytic therapies is what they call 'a real relationship between the two people doing therapy together which in our work is central to the reparative work'.[14] In discussing the 'real relationship' they emphasise the 'nurturing aspects of the therapist' in the process, an idea derived from Guntrip, 'which allows the client to take in and *embody* [my emphasis] the nurturing aspects of the therapist'.[15] By nurturing they seem to mean the 'process of feeling that the little girl is accepted, understood and *loved*

[my emphasis] by the therapist [which] is an extremely important aspect of the healing process'.[16] Now what is emphasised
here are the qualities that they think that the therapist *should*
bring to the situation. They also expect that

> The therapist *should* be open to talking about her theoretical
> biases, her prejudices and how her theory and practice view
> the psychology of women so that the client is aware of what
> sort of therapy she is committing herself to. All therapies
> are informed by a political perspective . . . Many psycho-
> therapists often make the mistake of offering us their work
> as if it were value-free.[17] (my emphasis)

Questions of love and beliefs are of course central to the problem of psychoanalysis. Nevertheless, the solution cannot be
prescriptive. There are very complicated issues at stake here
and in the end Eichenbaum and Orbach repeat the very
patterns that they set out to criticise. Their aim is to undo the
internalisation of women's oppression, but their theory leads
them in the direction of replacing one set of beliefs with
another. That is to say, a theory of a 'nurturing' therapist,
who can satisfy needs. There are problems here. The idea of a
nurturing therapist who can satisfy needs may reinforce a wish
for an ideal mother and lead to the client taking on the therapist's views and beliefs as a part of sustaining such an ideal.
In such a situation issues of love and belief may be left
unquestioned, not only for the client, but also in terms of
addressing what their functions are in mental life. Love is not
only about nurturing and mother-love; it is also about passions.
It is here that the crucial question of what is 'real' arises. There
are, of course, real elements always at play, the problem being to
determine what they are. Eichenbaum and Orbach believe that
they can be separated from the question of fantasy, and that the
distinction between the inside and the outside is also a relatively
straightforward one. Transference, they say, is not 'a very complicated phenomenon . . . It is the phenomenon of bringing
one's emotional responses from the past, the ones that we have
acquired from childhood, into everyday life.'[18]

These questions can, I think, be summarised under two
headings:

1. *How* the values and assumptions of the therapist affect the therapy situation, and particularly the client. This raises another question about *what* it is of the external world that affects the inner psychological world, and how these experiences are taken into the inner world.

2. What is the aim of therapy? For Eichenbaum and Orbach, for example, it would appear to be a re-mothering in the sense of compensating and making good what the client was deprived of in her childhood; that is, a consistent experience of being 'loved' and 'understood'.

There are certainly other important questions addressed by Eichenbaum and Orbach in their book, but these two are theoretical problems that also raise questions about therapeutic technique.

Psychoanalysis from its very beginnings has been struggling to illuminate the link between the internal and external – the effect the internal brings to bear on the external, and vice versa. In Freud's writings the question is never far away. It can be seen very clearly in his early theory of the seduction of the child by a parent, and his subsequent discarding of this in favour of the priority of the Oedipus complex, and the importance of fantasy. He struggled with the problem all his working life and did not resolve it. In discarding the theory of seduction, Freud was not saying that the external world is irrelevant, or that parents never seduce their children. He knew that some did. What he was trying to do was to understand what was being communicated to him in his consulting room through his patients' symptoms and their history. He wanted to know how his patients made sense of external reality. For Freud, external reality is not taken in whole, but in bits and pieces, which then need to be mentally digested. Many of the developments since Freud have lost sight of this question of the place of the external in the inner world of the individual. It is a question of utmost importance for feminists and one that was brought to the fore again in their challenging of women's position in society.

The women's movement has been heavily critical of the nuclear family, seeing it as an institution wich perpetuated the oppression of women. Orthodox analysis was criticised for not questioning the dominance of the nuclear family, and for designating mental health as coterminous with a satisfactory nuclear family life. In so far as there is truth in such criticisms, then some psychoanalysis can be seen to have become confused about the link between the internal and the external. The aim of psychoanalysis cannot be thought about primarily in terms of external phenomena, because it addresses internal processes. Anybody who is dissatisfied with the prevailing social reality and wants to change it needs a theory not only of how the external enters into the inner world, but also of what in the external has consequences for the internal.

Eichenbaum and Orbach take the link between the internal and the external to be very direct, and this results in confusion. On the one hand, for example, they say:

> Women discovered that they shared feelings of powerless-
> ness and rage, a sense of themselves as less than whole
> people, of frustration and underdevelopment; they had
> common experiences of being led into specific roles and
> activities, of being discriminated against, of being limited in
> sexual expression . . . [19]

The reality of having 'a sense of themselves as less than whole people' is taken as straightforward – in a certain sense real. However, women who have 'romantic or passionate feelings are not taken at face value, but are scrutinised for clues to understand their derivation and to grasp why such feelings are so important in the individual and collective lives of women'.[20] This reality is questioned. How do they get into this position where some statements are questioned and others not?

In the Introduction to *Outside In . . . Inside Out* they write: 'A feminist psychotherapy is interested in *how* the social prac- tices of a given culture are transmitted to its members and *how* the individual internalises the power relations, the sex-roles and the psycho-dynamics of the family' (my emphasis).[21] But later on they say 'we rejected a view of "self" conceived outside cul- ture and began to see how individual reality and personality is shaped by the material world. We see the unconscious as the intra-psychic reflection of our present child-rearing and gender relations.'[22] In this last sentence they defuse the radical nature of their enquiry by making the internal a reflection of the external. And although they are aware that it cannot be like this, they none the less write as though it is.

Eichenbaum and Orbach accept as a fact that women's sense of themselves as 'less than whole' is not only a true expression of an experience, but also a true statement about people: namely, that some people are 'whole' and presumably these people are men; it is after all women who are 'second-class'. They then elaborate a theory on the basis of this. They emphasise deprivation which they believe is primarily experienced by the little girl: women, in their view, suffer from inadequate and erratic mothering, because of the mother's identification with her girl child. They think that this is qualitatively worse than what is experienced by the little boy and that the girl child takes in, therefore, a worse experience. They believe however that it is potentially reparable, particularly in therapy. If the deprivation is re-experienced and worked through in the therapy, then with the therapist's re-mothering the client can make good her loss and thereby develop a sense of herself as a whole person. From this they can then argue that if we can change the little girl's early experiences then they too can become whole people from the start. External reality can thus in time be changed to create a new and rosier world.

The psychoanalytic tradition that Eichenbaum and Orbach draw on is that which is sometimes called 'object-relations theory', in particular the work of Fairburn, Guntrip and Winnicott. Their reading of these writers enables them to give an account which, at least from their point of view, produces a theory which adequately accounts for the social conditions that perpetuate the position of women as second-class citizens. None the less, they remain critical of object-relations theory, since they argue that it objectifies the mother and fails to understand that the 'mother is a person, a social and psychological being'.[23] This is in contrast to a point emphasised by Kohon with respect to these theories:

> The theory concerns itself with the relation of the subject to his objects, *not* [Kohon's emphasis] simply with the relationship between the subject and the object, which is an interpersonal relationship . . . It is not only the real relationship

with others that determines the subject's individual life, but the specific way in which the subject *apprehends* [my emphasis] his relationship with his objects (both internal and external). It always implies an unconscious relationship to these objects.[24]

In emphasising 'mother is a person', Eichenbaum and Orbach fail to take account of the unconscious.

In discussing Freud they accept his observation that women feel inferior, but they reject his explanation of the Oedipus complex and penis envy. They say:

This sense of inferiority is not formed at the Oedipus stage when the little girl realises she is not a boy; it is intimately linked to the very beginning of a girl's life and the acquisition of her gender identity. This sense of gender is woven into the very fabric of earliest experience: infants are related to as girls or as boys with all that attends those terms. When a woman reveals that she feels unsatisfied, inadequate, empty she is talking about her internal experience of being a woman in our society. These feelings arise because the psychic sphere reflects that she is a woman in patriarchal culture and a second class citizen.[25]

Eichenbaum and Orbach lose sight of the point made by Dinnerstein that human development is prompted through loss, and that life thereafter will always be a deeply ambivalent experience. They argue that a woman's sense of dissatisfaction and inadequacy is a consequence of inadequate mothering. If we take Dinnerstein's point, there is a sense in which the child's experience of its caretakers – male or female – is always going to be experienced as insufficient or inadequate. Eichenbaum and Orbach concentrate on 'need'. A little girl fails to get her needs met, when by implication little boys do. As we shall discuss in the next section, Mitchell shows that needs can never be known purely in themselves. They are known only through their relation to pleasure–unpleasure; the infant suckling at the mother's breast is not only satisfying a need, but experiencing something sensually pleasurable, which sets it off on its journey of differentiation. Satisfaction can only be temporary

– if it were permanent human beings would have no mental life – so whether or not the little girl has really been deprived by her mother, she is going to experience her mother's absence as a deprivation. Eichenbaum and Orbach hoped to show that the difference between the sexes is purely a socio-cultural phenomenon. The problem is, of course, that though there is an external world which does affect the inner life of all human beings, aspects of internal life that are not directly dependent on the existing outside world also affect the position of women.

Psychoanalysis and Feminism

I now want to consider a third writer who has used psychoanalysis as a way of contributing some insight into the relation between the individual and society, with respect to feminism. Juliet Mitchell wrote *Psychoanalysis and Feminism* in the early 1970s and it was published in 1974. This book is very rich in thought but here I am concentrating only on certain aspects of her work on Freud. Her reading of Freud is very influenced by the work of Jacques Lacan and the way in which his work was taken up by a number of Marxist feminist groups based in Paris and called *Psychanalyse et Politique*. They were, she says, 'part of the movement that has been trying consistently for some time to turn psychoanalytic theory into political practice – to raise both the general question of patriarchal ideology and the detailed issues of feminine psychology'.[26]

Mitchell's position appears to be very pessimistic with respect to political change, since it offers no solutions. Towards the end of the book she says:

> In brief, the thesis of this book is to know the devil you have got . . . We have a culture in which, with infinite complexity, the self is created divisively, the sexes are divided divisively; a patriarchal culture in which the phallus is valorized and women oppressed. Long before a situation is analysed, people wish for its overthrow . . . [27]

For many feminists, Mitchell's work is also highly disturbing because she seems to return to the very problems that many women have wanted to throw out as no longer relevant, or have dismissed as anti-feminist formulations. However, it seems to me that many of Mitchell's arguments are very compelling and point in a direction which is neither beset by ideals, nor insists on imposing a certainty of meaning upon the subject's life or on explaining it on the basis of biology. At the heart of her work is the idea that central to the problem of the relation of the individual to society is the predicament that we are thinking, speaking, desiring beings driven to make sense of our lives and desires. So we have to understand *how* we make sense of ourselves in the world and *how* we make sense of the world in which we are living if we are to come to an understanding which could be productive for the future.

Like Dinnerstein, Mitchell posits a dissonance between the individual and society. However, where Dinnerstein believes the gap can be and needs to be closed, Mitchell understands the dissonance as fundamental to human social life – an asymmetry, which cannot be eliminated (see p.247 above). In Freud, neurosis is a condition of civilisation, because there is an inescapable conflict between individual desires and social demands and needs. There is something anarchic in the nature of sexuality, which can never be entirely subdued by the human social order. Mitchell's view is that our relation to external reality is always a problematic one, because our understanding of it is filtered through our individual psychological inner worlds. The way in which we make sense of ourselves in the world is constructed through what we have taken in from the external world. However, what we take in is not just a reflection of the external, rather it is fragmented and refracted, and we have to put it together and order it within ourselves so as to make sense of it. There is of course an external reality, which is not a figment of our imaginations, and which we cannot take for anything we fancy, but at the same time, for each of us, our access to that reality is mediated by fantasy. Freud's theories are about *how* we acquire thought structures and *how* we come to make sense of our individual lives. As he discovered, this does have implications for society.

Freud's discoveries and his theories came mainly from his

work with adults in the consulting room. His theories of the mind are constructed through this work. They refer back to the patient's childhood because it is in these formative years that the structures and processes of the mind through which we make sense of our lives are constructed. But this is not a developmental account in the sense of privileging a certain sequence. (There are certain things which happen sequentially, and this was a problem that Lacan was later to analyse in terms of structure.) Freud compares it rather to archaeology, and like archaeology the discoveries come in fragments needing to be reconstructed. However, he believes it is none the less scientific.[28]

His first and most crucial discovery was the deduction of the unconscious. Freud does not have a unified theory of the unconscious; he gave at least two different accounts of it over the years he was working. They are not entirely compatible, but neither are they mutually exclusive. Freud hypothesised the unconscious because he came to realise, initially through his work on hypnosis, and later after discarding hypnotic techniques, that his patients knew more about themselves than they were consciously aware of. Their hysterical symptoms seemed to be the physical expression of a mental conflict, involving ideas that were debarred from consciousness. He soon discovered other symptoms of the unconscious: dreams, slips of the tongue, jokes, etc. All these were a means whereby the unconscious could express thoughts and ideas that could not be admitted to consciousness.

> The unconscious that Freud discovered is not a deep, mysterious place, whose presence, in mystical fashion, accounts for all the unknown; *it is knowable and it is normal* . . . normal thought utterly transformed by its own laws (what Freud called the primary process), but nevertheless only transformed hence still recognizable if one can deduce the manner of the transformation, that is, decipher the laws of the primary process to which the thought is subject.[29]

At the same time Freud discovered that what he came to call fantasy was fundamental to the thought processes of patients. Hearing again and again his patients tell him that they had

234 Living with the Sphinx

been seduced by their fathers in childhood originally led Freud to formulate the hypothesis that 'the repressed memory of actual childhood incest was reawakened at puberty to produce the neurosis'.[30] What he then discovered was a fantasy structure – a repressed wish on the part of the child that incest take place: however, it is a childhood wish formulated in adult speech. As Mitchell emphasises, Freud's concern here is with a mental process: as Freud knew, '*actual* paternal seduction or rape occurs not infrequently'.[31] There is, however, something else at stake here, which it is also important to explore: that is, the structure of a wish. The question of this structure is also explored by Freud in his analysis of dreams, symptoms and hallucinations.

The child's wish is of a different order from adult sexuality; for the child it is a crucial component in the construction of becoming a thinking, speaking, desiring and sexed human being. From there Freud went on to formulate his theories of infantile sexuality and later the Oedipus complex, which show how a child's conception of incest cannot be the same as that of an adult. What he makes clear is that the task of the adult is to maintain a taboo on incest.

The baby born of human parents has only a potential for human beingness. It does not yet have a mind – that is to say, it has no mental structures with which to make sense of its experiences. In order for it to become a human being the baby and the caretaking environment have to struggle with each other. Not only with each other, but also with themselves. In the struggle mind is born for the baby, and the possibility for meaning is kindled. It is a struggle that goes on until death. There is no easy relation between the inner psychological world of the individual, and social life. The human subject is constructed through conflict both within itself and with the environment. There is consequently no unified subject, and even an integrated subject is fragile. The subject's history is constantly open to reconstruction, since we give meaning to our experiences retrospectively and construct our knowledge and understanding of ourselves in the light of this retrospection. This is one of the radical discoveries of psychoanalysis. Such reconstruction is what allows the possibility for change.

Life and psyche are always potentially in motion, our understanding being taken apart, constructed, and reconstructed in the process. The baby – and child – has to engage with the demands of culture if it is to become a human being. At the same time each baby that is enabled to make this hazardous and 'tortuous' journey also pays a price, since each new move also involves a loss of the sense of self that was before.

As we saw above, Mitchell emphasises a reading of Freud which is not developmental as such. (There are, nevertheless, implications for developmental accounts in his work, and Freud was sufficiently ambivalent about the problem of development to accept Karl Abraham's theory of stages.) There are things which the infant–child experiences sequentially e.g. breast-feeding, potty-training, and recognition of sexual difference, which affect the mental structures from which it constructs a sense of itself. The point that Mitchell makes is that these stages are like stations in a journey, in which the next stop puts into a new perspective that which has gone before and which is therefore retrospectively understood in a new light, even though aspects of the previous structure remain.

I shall now give an account of the Mitchell baby in certain aspects in an attempt to indicate how the external does intrude in such a way as to ignite and structure the inner psychological world of the infant and young child. It maps out the mental terrain which enables the child to enter human culture. It should be understood that I am introducing this notion of a baby as a metaphor, which attempts to illustrate some of the problems I am discussing here.

This infant has no notions of self and otherness for some time. The first differentiation it makes is pleasure–unpleasure. Freud does not think that relationships with others are 'natural' even though they are necessary if the baby is to survive; it is through the infant's experiences of its own body and the experiences of pleasure–satisfaction and unpleasure – dissatisfaction that the baby initially comes to be able to situate itself in the world. He postulates several mental processes that are invoked by the infant to keep at bay the painful–unpleasurable experiences of the external world: human beings find external reality extraordinarily painful to deal with right from the start and have the capacity to retreat from it.

The baby's first internal mental process is the capacity to hallucinate – particularly the absent breast.[32] Of course, a hallucinated breast cannot satisfy hunger and so the hallucination fails and the baby experiences real deprivation. It is this real deprivation that intrudes and initiates the baby's journey into becoming a human subject.

The human subject is constructed through 'component drives' which are themselves constructed from bodily functions such as feeding, defecating, urinating, etc., and bodily senses such as seeing, hearing, feeling, etc. These drives are only known through their mental representations – that is, the idea that one constructs of something within the working through of the process of differentiation from others. They can never be known in themselves apart. The subject's experience of its body is mediated through the psychical processes by which it comes to make sense of itself and its experiences in the world. In this way need cannot be known independently either; for Freud there is always need plus something else. The baby, for example, feeding at the mother's breast not only takes in the milk, but also has a sensual experience particularly in the area of its lips. This has the effect of erotogenising the lips and also of creating an awareness of a bodily edge or hole.

During its journey towards becoming a human subject, the baby will come to differentiate between – amongst other things – absence, loss, lack, something missing, want, etc. The point about these distinctions is that they are crucial to the structuring processes. Dinnerstein does not make the distinction between these different experiences which designate different sorts of gaps. Each experience will alter the pattern – like a kaleidoscope – sometimes slightly and sometimes structurally. The difference is that unlike a kaleidoscope the old structures will remain and can be reactivated.

How does this infant come to recognise and differentiate the other? The first indication that there is something outside of it is the absent breast, which when lost seems to be a loss of the baby itself and potentially thrusts the baby into a disordered and undifferentiated state again. This initiates in the baby a search for itself, and the other is discovered in the process. The baby looks for itself in its mother's face. Where Winnicott emphasises the mother reflecting back to the baby its facial moods, Lacan emphasises a comparison – a difference. By contrast with the baby's lack of co-ordination, in the face of the other it finds what seems whole, harmonised. The baby, as yet unaware of a sense of itself as one, has experienced itself and its body as bits and pieces, unaware of how it all fits together, or even perhaps of what belongs to it – unutterably and helplessly dependent. The face in contrast and then whole people will appear as organised, co-ordinated. The moment in which the infant experiences itself as whole and co-ordinated is designated by Lacan 'the mirror phase'. This is the original identification of the ego, and the basis for all future identifications. This moment, which happens usually at between six and eighteen months is the moment when the infant recognises itself 'jubilantly' in the mirror. It beholds itself and assumes an internal image of itself as perfectly whole, co-ordinated etc. However, this recognition is imaginary, since the baby is still physically uncoordinated and helplessly dependent. The crucial point is that this first sense of itself means that the construction of the ego – as opposed to the subject – is founded in a fiction and always will be. Consequently the infant–child's comprehension of another is marked by the fictional quality of this original identification.[33]

As we have seen, the baby's first indication that there is something outside itself is derived from the failure of its hallucinations and the experience of real deprivations. This capacity to hallucinate is the prototype of fantasy. The child's first identification – the moment of 'the mirror phase' – is based upon the perception of another; that is to say, its perception of its caretaker, or the image of itself in the mirror supported by its caretaker. This identification is another aspect of fantasy. We can see here how elements of the external world are taken in – not as a reflection – but actively re-ordered. Mental processes such as the mirror phase enable the infant and child to make sense of its experiences. The baby starts out by attempting to sustain itself as the world, the centre of the world, and so on. This narcissistic position Freud refers to as 'His Majesty the Baby'. It is through the defeats that the baby encounters with other people in its attempts to sustain its position that the infant begins to construct a sense of otherness. One of the important points of Freud's work is that for the child a recognition of 'otherness' as opposed to perceiving the other as an aspect of oneself is extraordinarily difficult to acquire, and just as difficult to sustain in a consistent way. On the one hand, the infant – child invents all sorts of ways of sustaining its narcissistic sense of perfection and wholeness; on the other hand, if it is not to stultify and is to be able to participate in human society, it has to move on. For, like Narcissus in the myth, if it did not the baby would remain fixed in its image.[34] So, in order to escape from this bondage, the baby has to move from a state of self-love only to a capacity to love others as well. But this is no altruistic love; it is based on a desire to live, to enjoy. 'It is a fundamental psychoanalytical thesis that a person will never wholly give up what he has once enjoyed.'[35]

In his paper 'On Narcissism', Freud states that there are two different classes of love-object choices. One is founded in the infant's narcissistic self-love, and the other in the parents' functions of loving and caring for the child. What is interesting is that a parent's love of its child is founded in the quality of the parent's own narcissism: 'Parental love, which is so moving and at bottom so childish, is nothing but the parents' narcissism born again, which, transformed into object-love, unmistakably reveals its former nature.'[36] (This spiral of parental narcissism, infant–child narcissism, and the necessary subjugation of the child's narcissism, Lacan later developed into theories on the nature of desire and the construction of the subject. This provides more clues towards an understanding of the link between the individual and society.) It is this point in Freud – that love is constructed through self-interest – that many post-Freudians rejected, preferring to think of the infant as other-directed, and therefore potentially altruistic.

How then does the shift from a narcissistic mode of thinking to a capacity for sustaining the difference between self and other come about? For Freud it is through the negotiation of the Oedipus complex and the identifications constructed in the process, together with the consequences of comprehending sexual difference. This allows the child to participate in social relations with some understanding of the function of fantasy: the process involves what Freud presents as the theory of castration complex – which is represented by Jacques Lacan as a theory of symbolic castration. The theory of castration is Freud's most controversial theory for many feminists. His work in this field follows the twists and turns of his theories and it is impossible to explore all the implications and complexities here. I give only a few clues to show the way in which this is a key process.

The Mitchell baby is disposed towards bisexuality. It has no sense of sexual difference, since it has no internal mental structures with which to think about such things. This is why I refer to the baby—child as an 'it'. Mitchell's reading introduces sexual difference as a vital mental process – part of the structuring process of the mind. In the narcissistic thought structures there is only a partial comprehension of 'otherness' since the other is perceived through a sort of punctured wholeness. At this point Freud is convinced that the child can only grasp the idea of one sort of genital. It cannot conceptualise in any meaningful way the idea of two different genitals. For Freud a peculiarity of human beings is the diphasic character of sexuality. The first phase in which the 'component drives' are constructed from the sense the child makes of its body he calls 'polymorphously perverse' or the phase of 'infantile sexuality'. It is the Oedipus complex and the construction of the meaning of sexual difference that – through a lengthy period of conflict – shatters and transforms the narcissistic structures and reconstructs them, enabling the child to acquire a sense of 'otherness'. This brings to an end the time of 'infantile sexuality', and is followed by a period of latency when the child's sexuality is quiet. The second phase of sexuality is evoked by puberty and the physiological changes which accompany it. At this time the early conflicts engendered in the first years of the child's life are reactivated and the young adolescent finds herself or himself reworking them, but this time from the perspective of new knowledge gained at puberty. It is then, and then only, that the penis and vagina take on sexual meaning in an adult sense: a sense that includes a notion of relationships between adults. We can see then how understanding is always subject to reworking even though the archaic structures can remain active.

We will look in turn at the Oedipus complex and its resolution in the castration complex. Freud drew on the myth of Oedipus to explain the unconscious fantasy life he found at the basis of neurosis in his work with adults, as he struggled with them to understand their identifications and conflicts.[37] The Oedipus complex is the structuring process by which the infant–child is enabled to extricate itself from the trap of the mother–child duality. It allows the child to grasp the symbolic dimension to life which is essential if it is to become an active participant in society. 'The Oedipus complex is the *repressed* ideas that appertain to the family drama of any primary constellation of figures within which the child must find its place. It is not the *actual* family situation or the conscious desires it evokes.'[38] Mitchell emphasises the processes by which a child constructs its identities and how they affect its capacity to participate in social life. The repressed ideas appertaining to the family drama are built around experiences of the external world, but they are always marked by fantasy. They are put together by the child in the terms available to its inner mental life, driven by the search the child undertakes for itself. Of course, the processes are helped or hindered by its own particular family constellation, but not at a conscious level. It is, thus, not a matter of the child taking inside itself the prevailing order of the world, as if mirroring it.

Freud was always concerned with the effects of the external world upon the subject – how the external world 'intrudes' into mental life. In order for the child to enter into the symbolic dimension – that is to say, its cultural heritage – it has to internalise the incest taboo into its mental life in order to be able to relinquish its parents as love-objects. The incest taboo establishes the break-up of the mother–child dualism through the intervention of a third: this is usually, but not necessarily, the father. The father also provides the child with more material for its researches for understanding itself and widens the scope of possibilities for itself. There are two processes at play here: the intervention into the dualism, and what it is that the father provides; they can occur regardless of the actual father's presence or absence. I am less concerned for the moment with investigating the operation of these two processes, than with the content of the child's enquiries and how this material is constructed in a particular way. It is how babies are made that interests the child because, says Mitchell, underlying this curiosity are questions such as 'Who am I?' 'Where do I come from?' which bear on the child's search for itself. This will lead into the child's search for what it can become: a mother or a father; a man or a woman; a boy or a girl.

In this search for itself the child has to work out, as we have seen, the difference between self and other. Identification is a part of this process of separation, and Freud's theory of identification is complex.[39] There are three types and there is not the space to go into them here, so what I want to say is particularly schematic. In a certain sense identification is present from the beginning. So before exploring the implications of the Oedipus complex I want to give an indication of how a type of identification is present almost from the start. The infant's first position in what I am calling the narcissistic thought structure (often referred to as pre-oedipal) is as 'love-object' in relation to the mother. 'Freud points out how in the very first moments of an infant's life when it feels at one with the mother's breast, there can be no real distinction between object-love and identification.'[40] So here the identification is total: the child is the breastmother; the breastmother is the child. The point about this identification is that it is not internalised, as such; it is not quite inside, neither is it quite outside. Another kind of identification is the illusion of co-ordination – 'the mirror phase', the first internalisation. The Oedipus complex too enables the child to identify itself as separate from the other and to explore the differences, so the child can occupy in its imagination several different positions. For example, the child can want to get rid of its father, identify with him and take its mother as love-object; and it can also want to give her a baby. Or the child can want to murder – that is to say, get rid of – its mother, identify with her and want to be given a baby by the father. This applies to both boys and girls. In this drama there are in fact four positions the child can occupy in its mind: masculine-subject, masculine-object, feminine-subject, feminine-object. How does the oscillation between these positions settle down? Mitchell quotes from Freud's case history of Little Hans:

FATHER: But only women have children.

HANS: I'm going to have a little girl . . .

FATHER: You'd like to have a little girl?

HANS: *Yes, next year I'm going to have one* . . .

FATHER: But why isn't Mummy to have a little girl?

HANS: Because I want to have a little girl for once . . .

FATHER: Only women, only Mummies have children.

HANS: But why shouldn't I?

FATHER: Because God's arranged it like that.

HANS: But why don't *you* have one? Oh yes, you'll have one all right. Just you wait.

FATHER: I shall have to wait some time.[41]

So how does the child come to understand the difference between the sexes? For Freud knowledge comes about through loss, which always involves a restructuring. In this case, it is a loss of narcissism. The narcissistic structure which has necessarily been supported for the child by the external mother must now be lost if the child is to find a position in society which it can sustain. What Mitchell emphasises here is a lack. One of the things the child has to come to terms with is 'the notion of alternatives: if you have one, you cannot have the other, above all you cannot have everything.'[42]

Mitchell's infant is born into the Oedipal structure. Even before it is born it will have been given a symbolic place by the family. It will have been discussed, fantasised about, named, etc. It will have been planned for, or conceived accidentally, and so on. These thoughts about the baby will mark it and – known or unknown – play their part in the child's history, in terms of how the child comes to make sense of these elements. In this account the idea of the father is always present – even if he is physically absent, as in artificial insemination. The child will be born into a situation that it will hear about and have to make sense of in terms of a mother and a father. Mitchell's reading of the Oedipus complex is partially influenced by Lacan, who has taken and reworked Freud's theories of this and the corresponding notion of the castration complex. Mitchell differs from Lacan in that she makes central the incest taboo, and seems to take it literally, whereas Lacan does neither. The idea of the Father is for Lacan a symbolic function, which breaks into the imaginary wholeness of the mother-child dyad. This function of the Father is only gone into by Mitchell in so far as it is a component of the Oedipal conflict, whereas Lacan takes it further. Mitchell thinks that the function of the Father is linked with the upholding of the incest taboo, which according to Lévi-Strauss is the fundamental law of human culture. For Mitchell the function of the Father and the incest taboo are mental processes; the actual father can, however, stand in for the symbolic Father, as can anyone else who is designated to that position by the mother. That is to say, through the unconscious images she has of this symbolic Father, which will address the child at an unconscious level. The child's 'omnipotent' attempts to discover the desire of the mother and to satisfy it, give way to its positioning itself in terms of the law. However, this can only occur so long as the mother's desire is constructed in such a way that her desire is directed elsewhere than towards her child. In this situation the child will be enabled to become in its turn an adult capable of sustaining desire.

Mitchell's taking up of Freud's castration theory is also mainly influenced by Lacan. This reading emphasises a difference, which the child has to make sense of. It is a difference of another order to the loss of the breast as a part of itself – it is, however, just as *real*. This reality, that is to say, the biological differences between the sexes, fundamentally attacks the child's narcissistic thought structures. It is not a question of the child grasping the nature of the processes of reproduction. As Lacan says: 'In the psyche, there is nothing by which the subject may situate himself as a male or a female being.'[43] It is, however, a question of whatever representations the child has already acquired being called into play to explain this difference – and to do so within a structure already organised in part by the demands for dominance of the symbolic Law. For Freud, the child's genitals are privileged because of the bodily pleasures it derives from masturbation. While the child probably discovers this pleasure by accident, the pleasure soon becomes attached to the Oedipal fantasies. The idea of 'castration' is constructed by the child, says Freud, from the slightest of hints. It is here that girls and boys part ways.

For the little girl the discovery that she lacks a penis requires an explanation. In her mind she imagines that she once had one and lost it. This is a childhood theory and it is linked in her mind to her incestuous desires and masturbatory fantasies for the mother and father, and the invocation of the Law represented by the father. It creates in her, says Freud, 'penis envy'. This is a shorthand for a fantasy that the penis is 'a superior counter-part of her own small inconspicuous organ'.[44] So the omnipotent fantasy 'I am the centre of my mother's world', or 'my mother is the centre of my world' is replaced in the girl child by the fantasy which explains this decentring through inadequacy or devaluation, and as such constitutes a severe narcissistic wound.

The little boy is just as shocked as the little girl by her lack. It is a severe narcissistic wound for him too. Her lack he explains by a similar fantasy: that she once had one and lost it, and that his could be taken away too in retribution for his incestuous desires and masturbatory pleasures in line with the Law of the Father. In this sense the boy has also to submit himself to the idea of castration. However, it is a threat that will continue to haunt him for the rest of his life.

It takes some time for both the boy and the girl to realise that the mother also lacks a penis, and that all people who belong to the category of females are in this position. Then the consequences and the outcome are different for the boy and the girl – what Mitchell calls 'asymmetrical'. For the boy the realisation that the girl lacks a penis leads to a mammoth repression of his incestuous desires, and he renounces them. This process is sustained by the creation of a very severe and threatening authoritarian internal image, that Freud came to call the superego, and which constitutes an identification with the Father of the Law. There is however a consolation attached to it – the promise that one day the little boy will grow up, possess substitutes for the mother and himself in turn become a father.

The outcome for the girl is more complex, if she is to follow the 'normal' path to heterosexuality. She has to change her primary sexual object from a woman to a man. She does not renounce the mother in the way that the boy can. She turns against the mother 'through what seems like a fault in nature': for Freud this also requires later on a shift in the locus of pleasure from the clitoris to the vagina. This Mitchell emphasises is psychologically determined – like the component drives, the vagina can also become erotogenised. The girl, imagining that she has been castrated, turns away from her mother in disappointment and turns towards her father for consolation, wanting from him a baby. The idea of a baby represents for her the desire for what she unconsciously believes she has lost – the penis.

These theories of the Oedipus complex and castration highlight the gap between conscious and unconscious knowledge. There is a dissonance between what we seem to know at a conscious level and the sense we make of our experiences unconsciously. The structure of the unconscious is of a different order from that of consciousness. For example, castration in the unconscious order is, says Mitchell, 'a *nodal point* stretching backwards and forth from birth to death summarising within its instance the totality of loss' (my emphasis).[45] It finds a likeness, says Freud, in 'the basis of the daily experience of the faeces being separated from the body or on the basis of losing the mother's breast at weaning'. Linking it with death, he continues, 'but nothing resembling death can ever have been experienced . . . I am inclined therefore to adhere to the view that the fear of death should be regarded as an analogue to the fear of castration.'[46]

The idea of 'castration' is subject to the laws of the unconscious, and it is one of the structures through which the subject perceives its life – both backwards and forwards. Ultimately its structure is established through the recognition that what the mother wants the child cannot satisfy. Castration is not the same as loss of faeces or loss of the breast, but in retrospect these events are seen through the lens of the discovery of sexual difference and 'castration'.

For both boy and girl there thus exists the idea of castration, and with it an unconscious idea is constructed of the phallus: 'the very mark of human desire; it is the expression of the wish for what is absent, for re-union (initially with the mother).' It also 'mediates and breaks up the possibility of incest and the dyadic trap'.[47] The phallus initially symbolises the place of the father in the desire of the mother; it is then the symbolisation of the desire for all that is lost, for all that is lacking, and for the necessity of renunciation. The baby then becomes invested in the girl's mind with the phallus, in terms of her unconscious wish that she will recover in motherhood all that she has lost, including re-union with the mother. The phallus also symbolises the question of the Father: 'Why could this father not have a baby?' Little Hans was puzzled about this question (see p.41). 'Lacan points out that there are two things which can never really be known but are always recognised: death and the father's role in procreation. It is the place of the Father, not the actual father that is thus here significant . . . '[48] Only the mother knows for sure who the actual father is, and whoever he is there are also the mother's fantasies of a father, which will mark the child. In this complex problem of the question of the phallus it is important to mention that the phallus is not the penis. The penis is a bit of the body, while the phallus is a symbol: 'The phallus masks the lack and shows it and makes the lack thinkable.'[49]

For Mitchell, at the heart of the human dilemma is an ethical question. The capacity for human-ness may be something we are born with, but being born does not in itself guarantee our humanity. Values, assumptions, moral beliefs, etc., are constructed in the process of each person's search for herself or himself. They are part and parcel of our identities; our capacity to sustain ourselves in the face of what we meet in our lives is determined by the unconscious mental structures and processes that form us as human beings. The assumption of a sexed identity, which is prompted by the fantasy of castration, is a moment of fundamental importance in the construction of ourselves as human beings. It is at this point that girls and boys take up a different position in relation to the Law of the Father, the taboo against incest. Neither child may possess or be united with its mother, but the boy and the girl must find a different resolution, and henceforth boys and girls, and later men and women, will occupy the same world but perceive it through a different lens. The question of how moral life is constituted is therefore of fundamental importance to psychoanalysis – something Freud sensed very early on in his work. In 1897, writing to Fleiss, he said: 'Another presentiment tells me, though I already knew – but I know nothing at all – that I shall very soon uncover the source of morality.'[50]

The importance of Mitchell's reading of Freud is that she can countenance this question without producing a reading which imposes a moral or an ethical position on the individual. What she shows is how we become subjects with an ethical stance, not what that ethical stance will be – as does Klein for example. It is the negotiation of the Oedipus complex and the castration complex, and the sexual identity that is constructed in the process, that will determine whether or not this ethical position is sustainable and satisfying or whether it is incapacitating. Our sexual identities are not bound by our biological sex, but are constructed out of the way in which we come to make sense of ourselves as physical and emotional human beings in the world, in relation to others. Consequently, girls can sustain masculine identities and boys feminine identities. Sexual difference is sequentially the last element in the structure of the mind, but it reorders and reconstructs what has preceded it.

Freud did not equate health with normality. Writing to a distraught mother who had contacted him about her son's homosexuality, he said:

> By asking me if I can help you, you mean, I suppose, if I can abolish homosexuality and make normal heterosexuality take its place . . .

> What analysis can do for your son runs in a different line. If he is unhappy, neurotic, torn by conflicts, inhibited in his social life, analysis may bring him harmony, peace of mind, full efficiency, whether he remains homosexual or gets changed . . . [51]

Mitchell says of psychoanalysis that it is 'about the inheritance and acquisition of the human order. The fact that it has been used to induce conformity to specific social mores is a further abuse of it . . . '[52] In a footnote Mitchell gives her 'ideal' definition of mental health: 'health is the uninhibited quest for knowledge, mental illness the painful pursuit of secondary ignorance – a need not to know, though the knowledge will insist on making its presence felt'.[53]

She argues in *Psychoanalysis and Feminism* that we can use psychoanalysis towards an understanding of patriarchal culture – a necessary condition for any change. Freud's theories are taken here as an analysis of patriarchy, and she emphasises the importance of understanding his concepts within the theoretical context that has produced them. It is useless to extrapolate a concept and then criticise it, since this places the concept in a context that is entirely different and will, therefore, be likely to acquire a different meaning: 'thus in "penis envy" we are talking not about an anatomical organ, but about the ideas of it that people hold and live by in the general culture, the order of human society.'[54]

Psychoanalysis, then, inevitably raises questions about the relation between the individual and society. In looking further at this, Freud turned to the anthropologists of his time; Mitchell turns to Lévi-Strauss.

> Lévi-Strauss has shown how it is *not* the biological family of mother, father and child that is the distinguishing feature of human kinship structures. Indeed this biological base must be transformed if society is to be instituted . . . [The prohibition of incest] forces one family to give up one of its members to another family; the rules of marriage within 'primitive' societies function as a means of exchange and as an unconsciously acknowledged system of communication. The act of exchange holds a society together: the rules of kinship (like those of language to which they are near-allied) *are* the society. Whatever the nature of society – patriarchal, matrilineal, patrilineal, etc. – it is always men who exchange women.[55]

The kinship structure is the perceivable expression of the unconscious incest taboo. It is the junction point between the individual subject and society. However, there is between the individual and the society also an 'asymmetry': the Oedipus complex is not a reflection of these social structures.

Lévi-Strauss thinks that the incest taboo not only addresses parents and children, but significantly addresses sisters and brothers. Incest, particularly between peers, would create a vicious circle from which no culture could be established. (Mitchell discounts the popular belief that there is anything 'wrong' with incest, by which I take her to be referring to biology.) The kinship relations are structured by two functions. Women function as objects of exchange; men function as the Father of the Law, thereby ensuring the conditions by which the socio-cultural network can be sustained. Mitchell along with Lévi-Struass insists that women's function as objects is not in itself derogatory, and neither is men's function as Father of the Law necessarily superior. It is the value that culture places on them under patriarchy that constructs the meaning of these functions in this way. The point is that each function is essential for the continuance of cultural life, and in this reading there is no necessity for each function to be assigned specifically to one sex or the other.

We can see then that Mitchell's analysis of culture and the way in which the human baby is able to take up its position as a sexed human being in cultural life is not linked to the biological functions, even though it is through the child's exploration of these biological functions, amongst other things, that it comes to discover its identity. Mitchell again: 'It is . . . not on account of their "natural" procreative possibilities but on account of their cultural utilisation as exchange-objects (which involves exploitation of their role as propagators) that women acquire their feminine definition.'[56]

The nuclear family is heir to the kinship structures and is a particularly pernicious form of social life. It is a misleading structure because it appears to coincide with biology: it is taken as an ultimately rational expression of society. The ideology of the nuclear family mistakes masculinity for paternity and femininity for maternity, and thereby attempts to defuse the anarchic aspect of sexuality. An individual's biological sex guarantees nothing.

Mitchell's reading of Freud shows how identity is always a

construction and always tenuous. Freud's thesis that she develops – that unconsciously human beings only recognise one sort of genital – is a radical one since it opens up new ways of thinking. It shows us that there is something in the nature of humanity which escapes – escapes meaning and escapes understanding. In these theories there is something in the way of femininity which cannot be registered by the unconscious processes, which is linked with the fantasy of castration. One of the consequences of this is that women's relation to pleasure is different from that of men and it is something that men seem to fear in women, and have tried to subjugate. This theory has been rejected by some as anti-feminist on the grounds that it is a denial of our reality. However, I think this misses the point. This theory addresses questions to the processes of the unconscious – particularly the mental structures – and it is something that little boys as well as little girls have to struggle with and live with. The question of what it means to be a woman is different for each of us, even though the meaning is constructed through something shared in common: the question of femininity and the difference between the sexes. It is precisely because there is something in the nature of humanity that escapes determination that means that change is possible. Otherwise we would be doomed to repetition. In the prevailing order women represent the possibility of social exchange, but femininity, on the other hand, signifies the anarchic element which cannot be subjected by society, and which prompts change and transformation.

Conclusion

Dinnerstein thinks that life is intrinsically a painful affair, and that there is a continual necessity to negotiate loss – be it of the original oneness, of immortality, or of omnipotence. She thinks that women bear the brunt of this pain in present-day sexual arrangements. Eichenbaum and Orbach, influenced by Dinnerstein's thesis of sexual arrangements, concentrate on women's pain, but do not seem to think that pain – of a brutal nature – is intrinsically part of life, as does Dinnerstein. Consequently their hopes for a better life can be highly optimistic.

Mitchell differs from Dinnerstein and Eichenbaum and Orbach in that she thinks that there is something always potentially unstable in the mental life of the individual which has consequences for social relations. This something involves the question of the sexed identity of the subject and her relation to her desire. Freud tells us that: 'A strong egoism is a protection against falling ill, but in the last resort we must begin to love in order not to fall ill, and we are bound to fall ill, if in consequence of frustration, we are unable to love.'[57] Later on in this paper he says: 'Loving in itself, in so far as it involves longing and deprivation lowers self-regard; whereas being loved, having one's love returned and possessing the loved object, raises it once more.'[58] So we can fall ill then, both from loving too much and from loving too little. There is a problem here about the ambiguous nature of enjoyment, which any theory of change must, I think, take into account.

In starting the Women's Therapy Centre, Eichenbaum and Orbach addressed themselves to the question of women's pain and its links with society. In doing so they gave birth to an organisation which has not only thrived but has increasingly been able to take in new and very different ideas, and deal with the resulting conflicts. With hindsight, I would say that one of the implicit but important effects of Eichenbaum's and Orbach's work has been to address the question of analytic practice and technique. Since the way that these questions originally arose in the women's movement was centred around the question of the power and authority of the analyst, Eichenbaum and Orbach dealt with the issue by developing a 'feminist therapy'. As is often the way, in tackling one problem others get lost. In wanting to bring back into analytic thinking the importance of the external world, including the position of the analyst, which they thought had become forgotten, in my view they neglected the problem of fantasy life and the implications of this for the sexed subject. Eichenbaum and Orbach emphasise the real relationship between the therapist and the client. By real they mean (i) the real in the room including the transference and (ii) real in the sense of a genuineness between the therapist and client. In putting this emphasis and setting aside the function of fantasy in the therapy relationship, there is a danger that the therapist is set up as an ideal for the client.

Ideals of any sort are precisely what analytic therapy or analysis must put in question. Ideals are a means, among others, by which the subject in her fragility can sustain herself, by providing a support which creates an illusion of cohesion. In fear of annihilation or of collapse into chaos, human beings will harness values, assumptions, morality, etc., as such supports. They will also, in order to sustain themselves and in the name of a 'better life' demand that others identify with their beliefs. This can be lethal – not only for the individual, but also for society. An extreme example of this is fascism. This is not to say that ideals can or should be entirely given up, but that it is important to understand their function in mental life. This is why psychoanalysis and psychotherapy also have at heart a question about the nature of ethics.

Assuming an ethical position is not about making moral choices. It is what enables the subject to make such choices in the first place. An ethical position is taken up in relation to the subject's understanding of the fantasy of castration; it is the fantasy of castration which secures a split in the subject which can never be healed. This split is established at the time of the 'mirror phase'. From then on the child has to comprehend and manage the discrepancy between the fictional identification of wholeness or perfection and the disorder of its inner life. Submitting to a fantasy of castration – for both boy and girl – designates a lack, which is in effect a renunciation of something of the other sex, and therefore of the possibility for wholeness, completeness, perfection. Freud pinpointed this inescapable split when he disengaged the notion of heterosexuality from the domain of the 'natural', 'innate' or 'organic'. He showed that desire is constructed, and that the external object that can satisfy must in some way be able to sustain the subject's fantasy. This means that the individual's relationships with others are always marked by fantasy, and raises the question of what kinds of relationships are possible. What is put into question by this is how ethical positions are constructed and how some sort of morality is necessary for civilisation to be sustained. There are three problems which can be traced throughout Freud's work, and which are relevant here:

1. Articulated most explicitly in *Civilised Sexual Morality and Modern Nervous Illness* (1908) is the extent to which the demands of civilisation harm the subject, by imposing strict moral constraints upon her and making her neurotically ill, and which thus severely inhibit the possibilities for a satisfying life.
2. What moral demands are necessary for civilisation to be perpetuated?
3. Is there anything within the subject which eludes and perhaps contradicts the demands of civilisation?

Dinnerstein overcomes these problems by holding to a Kleinian theory. The Kleinian position is described well by Michael Rustin:

> I would summarize this body of work as offering a view of human beings which in an intense and unusual way *assumes* [my emphasis] them to be moral in their fundamental nature. It also, and in a close relation to this, assumes them to be constituted as social beings in a primary and continuing interdependency with others. Kleinian theory is impregnated with moral categories, and its developmental concepts – especially those of paranoid-schizoid and depressive positions – incorporate moral capabilities (notably of concern for the well-being of other persons) into their theoretical definition. A stage of development is partially defined in terms of the moral capacities typical of it. There is also an important revision of Freud's view of the moral sense in Klein's account of development especially in the distinction between persecutory and reparative guilt. Freud's superego is conceived as having a repressive and persecutory function, and Freudian analysis could therefore be understood as an emancipation from guilt, especially sexual guilt. In contrast, guilt in Klein's 'depressive position' is understood to arise from the recognition of the pain suffered by or inflicted on others, and as an essential part of relatedness. Capacity for moral feeling, therefore, in its more and less benign forms, is seen as a definable attribute which links human beings, rather than as an unfortunate external constraint upon them.[59]

Klein's work shifts the emphasis away from the question of the construction of sexuality, and therefore from questions of identity, to the infant and young child's relation with the mother. It thus attributes enormous power to the function of the mother, and it is this that Dinnerstein takes up, particularly because it appears to coincide with the external reality that women are the primary caretakers. Dinnerstein emphasises this function of mothering and introduces a very interesting idea about the effect of the mother's will and intention on her infant. Because she stays with Klein she cannot show *how* the mother's desires affect the baby, which is what she seems to want to do. This brings in the question of the unconscious and would lead in the direction of Mitchell's reading of Freud. As it is, Dinnerstein can only emphasise the external reality, that women are the primary caretakers, and she has to concentrate on proposing a change in the nature of childcare arrangements. Mitchell shows us how our understanding and sense of our body and our bodily sensations are a construction. In Klein, the baby is innately other-directed and so, in its mind, it is outside its body, so to speak; in order to account for how the infant makes sense of its bodily sensations Klein posits innate, pre-organised feelings, which seem to be the innate, concrete building blocks of human sense. Dinnerstein would seem to go along with this and as a consequence the individual's knowledge and understanding of her body seem to be relatively unproblematic. Sexual identity is not an issue.

Eichenbaum and Orbach, although they are particularly influenced by Dinnerstein, try to avoid a theory which depends upon an innate explanation. They do not, however, have an explanation of how a moral sense is constructed, or how it relates to sexual difference, and it is difficult to see why or how their vision of no difference could be sustained, even if all the difference in upbringing between little boys and little girls were to be eliminated. But also – and this is the crux of the matter – the subject is taken for granted. What gets lost is how it is constructed and it is this that brings us back to the question of sexual difference. For Freud, as Mitchell shows, the human subject is not, never has been, and never will be whole:

There is no nostalgic normality nor . . . any childhood bliss when all is as it should be. On the contrary, in childhood all is diverse or perverse; unification and 'normality' are the effort we must make on our entry into human society. Freud had no temptation to idealise the origins with which he was concerned.[60]

Central to any feminist pursuit is the question of individual and social change. Any such consideration has always to take account of human desire, either explicitly or implicitly. It is well known that social forces limit the possibilities for an individual in any culture; but what is more disturbing – particularly for the Left – is a consideration of whether or not there is anything endemic in the constitution of the human subject, which imposes constraints on us in establishing a 'better life'. (This point is also made by Rustin in the above-mentioned article.)

The human subject is split, and the subject's ethical position is taken up in relation to its capacity to tolerate this split. This is profoundly a question of desire. Mitchell's reading of Freud shows how problematic heterosexuality is and that its basis is linked not to the propagation of the species but to the continuance of civilisation, as organised around the notion of difference. This difference is sustained by the Law of the Father. In order to sustain civilisation – which is always a very tentative affair – and to change the patriarchal law, we have to find another way of implementing and sustaining difference. Eichenbaum and Orbach search for a way of life in which need could be satisfied. What is left out here, is that in order for us to participate in social life we can never just know need, and that if we were to live a life without desire or alternatively where our desires were fully met, we might just as well only play at being alive. Dinnerstein, who takes up seriously the question of passion, still hopes that it is a fairly straightforward matter – like the satisfaction of a need. What Mitchell shows us is that passion and desire constitute not only what is necessary to the human subject, but also the disruptive element in it.

Acknowledgments

I want to thank Sheila Ernst, Julia Vellacott, and Bernard Burgoyne, each of whom has made a difference to this article: it has benefited greatly from their contributions.

Vivien Bar

Notes

1. Butterfly to Captain Pinkerton, from Puccini, *Madam Butterfly*, John Calder, London, 1984, p.94.
2. This book has also been published under the title *The Mermaid and the Minotaur*. References in this article are to the edition published in 1978 by the Souvenir Press, London.
3. Penguin, Harmondsworth, 1982.
4. Penguin, Harmondsworth, 1986.
5. Dinnerstein, *The Rocking of the Cradle*, p.8. Dinnerstein is here (approvingly) paraphrasing from Norman O Brown, *Life Against Death*.
6. ibid., p.121.
7. ibid.
8. ibid., p.135.
9. ibid., p.133.
10. ibid., p.176.
11. Melanie Klein, *Envy and Gratitude and Other Works*, Hogarth Press and the Institute of Psycho-Analysis, London, 1984.
12. ibid., p.179.
13. Eichenbaum and Orbach, *Outside In . . . Inside Out*, p.11.
14. ibid., p.50.
15. ibid., p.62.
16. ibid.
17. ibid., p.69.
18. ibid., p.48.
19. ibid., p.11.
20. ibid., p.13.
21. ibid.
22. ibid., p.15.
23. ibid., p.113.

24. G. Kohon, 'The psychoanalytic movement in Great Britain' in
    G. Kohon (ed.), *The British School of Psychoanalysis*, Free
    Association Books, London, 1986, p.20.
25. Eichenbaum and Orbach, op. cit., p.107.
26. Juliet Mitchell, *Psychoanalysis and Feminism*, Penguin, 1986.
    p.xxi.
27. ibid., p.361.
28. For an account of science and Freud, see Juliet Mitchell, 'The
    question of femininity and the theory of psychoanalysis' in G.
    Kohon (ed.), *The British School of Psychoanalysis*.
29. Juliet Mitchell, *Psychoanalysis and Feminism*, p.6.
30. ibid., p.9.
31. ibid.
32. See Freud, *The Interpretation of Dreams*, The Standard
    Edition of The Complete Works of Sigmund Freud, Hogarth
    Press, London, 1975, vol. 5, p.565.
33. For an account of the development of the notion of the ego
    in Freud and in French psychoanalysis see the articles 'Ego',
    'Ego-ideal', and 'Ideal Ego' in J. Laplanche and J.-B.
    Pontalis, *TheLanguage of Psycho-analysis*, Hogarth Press,
    London, 1973.
34. For an account of the Narcissus myth see Mitchell,
    Psychoanalysis and Feminism, p.30.
35. ibid., p.34.
36. ibid. (quoting Freud).
37. For Freud's account of the Oedipus myth which is drawn from
    Sophocles' drama, see The Standard Edition of the Complete
    Psychological Works of Sigmund Freud, Hogarth Press, London.
38. Mitchell, op. cit., p.63.
39. See Freud, *Group Psychology and the Analysis of the Ego*,
    The Standard Edition of the Complete Works of Sigmund
    Freud, Vol. 18.
40. Mitchell, op. cit., p.70.
41. ibid., p.25. Mitchell quotes Freud's case history 'Analysis of a
    phobia in a five-year-old boy'.
42. Mitchell, op. cit., p.26.
43. J. Lacan, *Four Fundamental Concepts of Psycho-Analysis*,
    Penguin, Harmondsworth, 1979, p.204.
44. S. Freud, *The Standard Edition of the Complete Works of
    Sigmund Freud*, Vol. 19, p.252.
45. Mitchell, op. cit., p.76.
46. Mitchell, p.77 (quoting Freud On Narcissism.)

258   *Living with the Sphinx*

47. Mitchell, p.395; p.393.
48. ibid., p.391.
49. This point was made by Patrick Guyomard at a weekend of seminars at Sussex University in May 1986.
50. Freud, The Standard Edition of the Complete Works of Sigmund Freud, Vol. 1, p.253.
51. Mitchell, op. cit., p.11 (quoting Freud).
52. ibid., p.401-2.
53. ibid., p.11.
54. ibid., p.xvi.
55. ibid., p.370.
56. ibid., pp. 407-8.
57. ibid., p.33 (quoting Freud).
58. Freud, 'On Narcissism', *The Standard Edition of the Complete Works of Sigmund Freud*, Vol. 14.
59. M. Rustin, 'A socialist consideration of Kleinian psychoanalysis', *New Left Review*, No. 131, Jan/Feb 1982.
60. Mitchell, op. cit., p.17.

A note from Susie Orbach on Vivien Bar's discussion of *Outside In . . . Inside Out, Women's Psychology: A Feminist Psychoanalytic Account*

Vivien Bar raises three points that relate to important topics of discussion within psychoanalysis. These are (1) The nature of the relationship between the therapist and client, (2) The developmental pathway to differentiation, and (3) The role of nurturance within the feminist psychoanalytic therapy. Clarity on these issues is important because differences here lead to very real differences in the understanding of an individual's difficulties and the course and conduct of therapy.

The relationship that develops between the therapist and the client or the analyst and the analysand, how to talk about it, how to understand it, and its role within the therapy have been discussed extensively for the last 50 years. Within modern psychoanalysis,* the British School of Object Relations and the Kohutians in the United States have taken the relationship between the analyst and the analysand as a focus of the therapeutic work.[1] In other words, the therapy itself constructs a relationship which, while individual and unique to each therapy relationship, is at the same time circumscribed by parameters which define that relationship. What can be expected to occur within that relationship, the transference aspects of it, the treatment alliance, the unconscious wishes

---

* Modern psychoanalysis refers to the work of Post-Freudians including British Object Relations, Kleinians, Kohutians, Middle Group Analysts, Sullivanians and Winnicottians.

projected on to the therapist by the client, the defences that the client brings with her into the therapy relationship, and the aspects of the therapist that are brought into the therapeutic frame, together constitute a *real relationship* between the two people engaged in a therapeutic contact.

During the course of therapy, the relationship develops and changes. It is these changes, as they are observed and 'worked' on within the therapy relationship, that modify the psychic structure of the individual in therapy. Modern psychoanalysis does not jettison the notion of transference or the exploration of unconscious processes, for this is the very stuff of therapy. Rather it takes the therapy relationship as a *real relationship* in which these can be grappled with so that the defence structure can dissolve as the subjectivity, or 'sense of self', is felt to be strengthened and secured.

What feminists have added to this tendency within psychoanalysis is the consideration of the myriad of meanings of gender both within the therapy relationship and in the life of the analysand and the analyst. In other words, because gender is a fundamental way in which the individual knows her or himself and is apprehended by others,[2] it is necessary to address the meaning of gender within the therapy relationship. Many aspects of the therapy relationship, the transference aspects of it, the desire for understanding and the despair about receiving it, the negation of need of the therapist and the wish for holding, the love and fear of women and so on become illuminated as client and therapist explore the psychological implications of gender within the therapy relationship. A consideration of the shared gender of mother and daughter and its significance is one of the contributions that feminists have been making towards psychoanalysis, both at a theoretical level and in terms of the implications for the conduct of therapy.

The second point – what constitutes the developmental path to differentiation – is closely related to the first. Differentiation has been a contentious issue within psychoanalysis ever since the focus of much analytic work has shifted from oedipal to the very early object relations. Differentiation in its clinical /diagnostic sense – as opposed to its popular sense – only occurs with the

Notes

1. Jay R. Greenberg and Stephen A. Mitchell, *Object Relations in Psychoanalytic Theory*, Cambridge, Mass, 1983.
2. John Money & Anke Erhardt, *Man and Woman, Boy and Girl: The Differentiation and Dimorphism of Gender Identity from Conception to Maturity*, John Hopkins, Baltimore, Maryland, 1972.
3. D.W. Winnicott, 'Ego Distortion in Terms of True and False Self' in *The Maturational Processes and The Facilitating Environment*, Hogarth Press, London, 1965.
4. W.R.D. Fairbairn, *Psychoanalytic Studies of the Personality*, London 1952.
5. Harry Guntrip, *Your Mind and Your Health*, London 1970.

Susie Orbach

Notes on the Contributors

Vivien Bar works as an analytic psychotherapist, who is also a feminist. She works part-time at the Centre and part-time in private practice. She is a member of the Guild of Psychotherapists. Her article is an attempt to formulate a way of thinking about some of the differences amongst those of us who work at the Centre, and what these differences mean for her. It is also an expression of an ongoing interest in the relations of the individual and society, particularly in terms of the question of sexual difference and the implications of this for women.

Mira Dana was born in Israel to parents of Arab Jewish origin. She was conscripted to the airforce after leaving school. During her university years she worked with the veterans of the army and later in a psychiatric hospital with drug addicts. In 1979 she joined the WTC while working on a Master's degree in psychology. Since 1981 most of her work at the Centre has been with eating problems, introducing her to a certain way of thinking about women's psychology which has been useful in understanding issues for women around abortion. She works as a psychotherapist, and leads workshops and lectures in the UK and Europe.

Luise Eichenbaum and Susie Orbach are the co-founders of the Women's Therapy Centre in London and The Women's Therapy Centre's Institute in New York. Their interest is both in the clinical and theoretical advances that feminism has to contribute to psychoanalysis. Luise Eichenbaum now lives and works in New York, while Susie Orbach is based in London.

Sheila Ernst's interest in separation grew from working with women, clients at the Women's Therapy Centre, reading and discussing D.W. Winnicott in the Women's Therapy Centre Study group, and developing the therapeutic approach of Luise Eichenbaum and Susie Orbach. Her views on separation were also influenced by her experiences as a group member and conductor of group analytic groups. She is a member of the Institute of Group Analysis. She works as a psychotherapist at the Women's Therapy Centre and as a groupwork consultant in Hounslow Social Services.

Margaret Green was born in Cape Town, South Africa to Jewish immigrant parents. She has a Master's degree in Biochemistry from the University of Cape Town. She lived for a time in New York before coming to London where, in 1971, she joined one of the early consciousness-raising groups of the women's liberation movement. Switching career was only one of the many resultant changes. In 1976 she joined the staff of the Women's Therapy Centre after it had been in existence for six months. Aside from being in private practice as a psychotherapist, she has led workshops on topics such as racism, classism, incest, Jewish identity and issues around colonisation and leadership.

Marie Maguire's involvement in this book has enabled her to bring together her interest in writing (which led her to study literature at university), her feminism and her work as a psychotherapist. Her previous jobs include working as a counsellor at a community mental health centre (Battersea Action and Counselling Centre). At the Women's Therapy Centre, where she has been a staff-member since 1980, she sees individual clients and teaches courses. She has a private practice and is a member of the Guild of Psychotherapists.

Carole Sturdy spent the late sixties and early seventies, after university, 'dropping out', working in a variety of temporary manual jobs in London while being active in libertarian left-wing groups such as the Claimants' Union, squatting groups, the Red Collective, as well as the women's movement. She has worked for the WTC and been in individual therapy for four years. She is thirty-nine and lives in North London with her ten-year-old son.